Texts in Applied Mathematics **10**

Texts in Applied Mathematics

Frank C. Hoppensteadt
Charles S. Peskin

Mathematics in Medicine and the Life Sciences

With 73 Illustrations

Springer-Verlag
New York Berlin Heidelberg London Paris
Tokyo Hong Kong Barcelona Budapest

Frank C. Hoppensteadt
College of Natural Science
Michigan State University
East Lansing, MI 48824-1115
USA

Charles S. Peskin
Courant Institute of Mathematical Sciences
New York University
New York, NY 10012
USA

Editors

F. John
Courant Institute of
 Mathematical Sciences
New York University
New York, NY 10012
USA

J.E. Marsden
Department of
 Mathematics
University of California
Berkeley, CA 94720
USA

L. Sirovich
Division of Applied
 Mathematics
Brown University
Providence, RI 02912
USA

M. Golubitsky
Department of
 Mathematics
University of Houston
Houston, TX 77004
USA

W. Jäger
Department of Applied
 Mathematics
Universtität Heidelberg
Im Neuenheimer Feld 294
6900 Heidelberg, FRG

Cover art by Charles S. Peskin and Peter H. Carrington.

Mathematics Subject Classification: 92-01, 92B05, 92D99

Library of Congress Cataloging-in-Publication Data
Hoppensteadt, F. C.
   Mathematics in medicine and the life sciences / Frank C.
Hoppensteadt, Charles S. Peskin.
      p.   cm. — (Texts in applied mathematics)
   Includes bibliographical references and index.
   ISBN 0-387-97639-6 — ISBN 3-540-97639-6
   1. Biomathematics.   2. Population biology — Mathematics.
3. Physiology — Mathematics.   I. Peskin, Charles S.   II. Title.
III. Series.
   [DNLM 1. Biology — methods.   2. Mathematics.   3. Models.
Biological.   4. Physiology — methods.   QT 35 4798m]
   OH323.5.H67   1991
   574'.01'51 — dc20
   DNLM/DLC
   for Library of Congress   91-4945

Printed on acid-free paper.

Photocomposed copy prepared using LaTEX.
Printed and bound by R.R. Donnelley & Sons, Harrisonburg, VA.
Printed in the United States of America.

9 8 7 6 5 4 3 2 1

ISBN 0-387-97639-6 Springer-Verlag New York Berlin Heidelberg
ISBN 3-540-97639-6 Springer-Verlag Berlin Heidelberg New York

Series Preface

Mathematics is playing an ever more important role in the physical and biological sciences, provoking a blurring of boundaries between scientific disciplines and a resurgence of interest in the modern as well as the classical techniques of applied mathematics. This renewal of interest, both in research and teaching, has led to the establishment of the series: *Texts in Applied Mathematics (TAM)* .

The development of new courses is a natural consequence of a high level of excitement on the research frontier as newer techniques, such as numerical and symbolic computer systems, dynamical systems, and chaos, mix with and reinforce the traditional methods of applied mathematics. Thus, the purpose of this textbook series is to meet the current and future needs of these advances and encourage the teaching of new courses.

TAM will publish textbooks suitable for use in advanced undergraduate and beginning graduate courses, and will complement the *Applied Mathematical Sciences (AMS)* series, which will focus on advanced textbooks and research level monographs.

Preface

Mathematical Biology is the study of medicine and the life sciences that uses mathematical models to help predict and interpret what we observe. This book describes several major contributions that have been made to population biology and to physiology by such theoretical work.

We have tried to keep the presentation brief to keep the price of the book as reasonable as possible, and to ensure that the topics are presented at a level that is accessible to a wide audience. Each topic could serve as a launching point for more advanced study, and suitable references are suggested to help with this. If the underlying mathematics is understood for these basic examples, then mathematical aspects of more advanced life science problems will be within reach.

The techniques presented here range in mathematical difficulty up to calculus and matrix theory. The material is presented in general order of increasing mathematical difficulty. Some exercises deal with material in preceding sections, others are projects that extend preceding material.

Our purpose in this book is not the systematic presentation of mathematical material, although there are important threads that run through several chapters. Instead, we hope to illustrate how mathematics can be used. In particular, our goal is to make available to students, having at least one term of calculus, topics in the life sciences and medicine that have benefited from mathematical modeling and analysis. In addition to exposing students to current ideas, the material is intended to reinforce their mathematics education by presenting familiar mathematical topics from novel points of view. Finally, enabling students to think in terms of models early in their academic experience should motivate them to develop and apply modeling skills further.

While hoping this interdisciplinary book will be useful to a wide variety of individuals, we believe that it can have special significance for the premedical student, who will find a mathematical introduction to a host of phenomena that are central to the practice of medicine. These include genetics and epidemics as well as the functions of the heart, lungs, and kidneys. It is our hope that the mathematical study of these topics will give the student a depth of understanding and insight that could not have been achieved through traditional, descriptive education in the medical sciences.

The mix of topics, taken largely from population biology and from physiology, includes important phenomena that are within reach of the students described above. The population part of the book draws its material from the areas of demographics, genetics, epidemics, and biogeography, while the physiological part surveys cardiovascular, pulmonary, renal, and muscle physiology. The final chapter is intended to introduce students to models of nerve cells and some neural circuits as a basis for studying how the brain works. We are on the rise of a wave of understanding of brain function, and mathematical modeling can be useful in understanding this complex organ.

We thank Anneli Lax for her early interest in the course that led to this book and for helpful discussion during the preparation of the lecture notes on which this book is based. Besides the authors, the course has been taught by Stephen Childress, H. Michael Lacker, and Daniel Tranchina, and we are indebted to them for their comments and advice.

Frank C. Hoppensteadt
Charles S. Peskin
November, 1990

Contents

Introduction

There are two major parts to this book. The first part (Chapters 1–4) introduces the mathematics of populations. This section begins with models based on iteration of reproduction curves; these can be done geometrically, with a hand calculator or with a computer. Starting with Malthus's model of geometric population growth and proceeding to models whose solutions are chaotic, we introduce various mathematical methods for studying and simulating model systems. Other topics include age structure and infinitesimal sampling intervals. The second, third, and fourth chapters are shorter than the first, and they are separated only because they study quite separate population phenomena. These chapters introduce ideas of probability theory to model random events in populations. Random models and their non-random analogues are developed, and through the chapters we discover how the random and non-random models are related. Two problems from genetics are studied in Chapter 2, Chapter 3 is about two problems from epidemics, and Chapter 4 is about dispersal processes. The models in Chapter 1 do not account for random sampling effects in populations, but the examples in the next three chapters do. The intention is to expose students early to ideas of probability in modeling, to build random and non-random models of similar phenomena, and to understand how the two are related.

Random sampling occurs in many settings, for example if a person who is capable of spreading a disease enters a group of people susceptible to it, there may or may not be an effective contact between the infective and a susceptible. Contact is a sampling process. If the group is very small and not in close contact, the probability of spread of the disease is small. If the group is large and in close contact, the probability is near one, and random effects can be ignored.

The basic tool developed here for accounting for random sampling is the Markov chain. Markov chain models are derived in all three chapters, and they are compared to analogous non-random models.

Both the random and non-random models lend themselves nicely to simulation using either a hand calculator or a computer. Computers are attractive because they offer a great range of presentations of output. However, many of the tables in the first four chapters show how one can present results from hand calculator computations in interesting ways. The use of both calculators and computers is encouraged.

The second part of the book (Chapters 5–10) deals with models from physiology. We introduce models of various organs and body systems using elementary ideas from physics. A background in high school level physics is sufficient for this material. The biological material need not have been studied before since the essentials are summarized in the text.

These six chapters present several important but distinct physiological systems (heart and circulation, kidney, etc.) while introducing many of the essential terms and ideas used in modeling the physical processes of flow, advection, etc. The final chapter introduces some ideas about neurons and how they might be organized into neural circuits involved in our breathing and thinking. The goal is to introduce students to the use of mathematical methods in modeling biological systems by doing simple computations that have been used decisively in understanding how these systems work. In addition to introducing students to important topics in physiology and steering them toward further study of them, our approach is intended to reinforce mathematical skills by applying them in plausible situations.

The range of material is intended to make possible courses at the undergraduate level ranging from one quarter to a full year without a great deal of editing being required of the instructor and students. The exercises are graded in difficulty from those that help beginning students to those that challenge advanced undergraduates. Some sections are denoted by *. These require more mathematical preparation or a softer touch in teaching. They can be skipped, although we believe that the material in these sections is important to bringing certain topics to closure.

Using this material we have taught premedical students, biology students, mathematics and physics students, computer science and engineering students, and some business students. This material makes possible cross disciplinary courses that can be taught by one instructor or several who come from applied mathematics, physics, engineering, social science, agriculture or biophysics backgrounds.

Here are some sample courses

One quarter: Chapters 1–4; or Chapters 5–9.

One semester: Chapters 1, 5 and 10

Two quarters: Chapters 1–6; or Chapters 1–4 and 10

One year: The entire text.

We have suggested several projects that can be assigned to groups of students working as a team. For example, students can construct a neuron model circuit, derive the mathematical model of the circuit, simulate the model on a computer, and analyze it using methods of differential equations; or students can perform a variety of chemostat experiments; or conduct a project in the economics of exhaustible resources.

Explanations are brief in most cases, and the intention is to provide a wide range of material at a reasonable cost to the students while still providing enough information to enable them to complete the exercises at the end of each chapter and to start reading in the scientific literature. The exercises are an important part of the text since it is through them that the students get an opportunity to apply material in the text and to create new applications from those methods.

With additional work by the instructor, it is possible to spend an entire term on one or two chapters. For example, heart and circulation lead to a variety of clinical examples of disease, or beginning with Chapter 10, one can launch into a term's worth of work on brain modeling. The modular structure of the book allows flexibility in course design.

This book uses mathematical modeling throughout, and the reader should be aware that such models are always based on simplifying assumptions. Simplification in mathematical modeling is both a blessing and a curse. The curse is the partial loss of predictive power that comes from whatever lack of correspondence there may be between the model and the real world. The blessing is the insight that comes from the process of pruning away unnecessary detail and leaving behind only what is essential. When Euclid said "a line is that which has no breadth," he was not describing anything that exists in the physical world, but history has vindicated his somewhat artificial conception. Because this is an introductory book, the simplifications made herein are even more extensive than usual, so the reader should be warned not to regard the statements or equations of this book as being literal or exact descriptions of biological reality. The models presented here are in the nature of metaphors, and these metaphors will have served their purpose if they have helped the reader to see through the bewildering complexity of living systems to the underlying simplicity of certain fundamental biological processes and functions.

1

The Mathematics of Populations: Demographics

What are population problems? Here are some examples:

1. What will the population of the U.S. be in 10 years?

It is reasonable to look at the record of population growth in the past and extrapolate this information into the future to predict population size. In this mathematical procedure, parameters such as the birth and death rates are estimated using past records, and the population of the future is projected by solving a mathematical model.

2. How will this population be distributed among age groups?

The same extrapolation methods are used, but the model becomes more complicated when we account for age structure. Now the parameters to be identified from available data are age-specific birth and death rates. The solution of an appropriate mathematical model determines the population's future age distribution.

3. How are exhaustible natural resources best managed?

A resource, such as a bacterial culture or a fishery or a forest, must be managed to provide optimal production while at the same time protecting the resource from extinction. Legal, social, financial and moral questions almost always arise with management of natural resources. Here we avoid all but the relatively simple questions of calculating yields from exhaustible resources, and we describe consequences of various optimal harvesting policies. Even with this severe restriction, there are difficult problems since each resource is part of a complicated interdependent network. The mathematical tools introduced here give some guides to study the economics of ecological systems, and they illustrate potential glaring pitfalls in management policies. In particular, the resource population might be driven into chaotic dynamics that can lead to its collapse.

4. Do the results of genetic engineering pose a serious threat to our environment?

To answer this question, we must understand the ways genetic information can be inherited and how pathogenic agents can spread throughout a population.

Genetic inheritance has been studied by philosophers, theologians, biologists, and physicians for more than a century. Even now, this research is controversial. We restrict attention here to genetic inheritance of relatively simple traits in bacteria and humans. Mathematical techniques are useful to project what gene distributions will be in future generations. We discuss genetics problems in small populations (small plasmid pools) and in large ones where there are many participants.

5. Can the spread of a contagious disease be predicted?

Questions about the occurrence and control of epidemics are raised by the spread of bacteria and viruses. Disease dynamics are traditionally described in terms of the numbers of susceptibles and infectives. We first discuss disease propagation in small populations such as families, and then in large ones such as schools or cities, to gain useful insight into the mechanisms of disease spread and control. Economic considerations also come up in disease control; for example, if a vaccine is available for a particular disease, how would the population best be inoculated within the constraints imposed by time, staff, medical facilities, age-specific host susceptibility, and the presence of competing diseases?

6. Are insect infestations in crops predictable?

Study of the geographical distribution of populations is the key to answering this kind of question. There are many possible ways populations move through regions, and mathematical analysis has led to methods for describing them. We study a random walk model and eventually derive a diffusion approximation to it. The derivation of the diffusion equation from a random process can be applied to the genetics and epidemics examples as well, and with this we see how the small population and large population models are related.

Why study these problems?

The impact on human populations of these problems is immense. For example, infectious diseases account for a staggering number of lost work days, uninhabitable geographical areas, and incapacitation and death of humans, animals, and crops. In addition, it is useful to understand our environment and to estimate risks to it. Calculations like the ones described here are routinely used by medical and public health planners, genetic counselors, industrial, community, and economic planners, and insurance providers, to name a few.

Mathematical methods in population biology can account for randomness, but it is not always necessary. As we have seen, these cases are separated by the population size. (Typically, a population is large if it has more than 30 members.) When a population is large, then random effects are not usually significant, and some complicated features of the population can be uncovered without great difficulty. When the population numbers are small, then random effects are very important, and it is necessary to calculate in detail possible changes in population numbers and how likely they are. Large populations often have a single most likely evolution, but small ones have many possible evolutions that have comparable likelihoods, and all of these must be described. We study large populations in this chapter, and in Chapters 2, 3, and 4, we compare models in small and large populations.

In this chapter we model population dynamics in a variety of settings. Predicting total population size, and even counting a population now, are difficult projects. They are made more complicated by the fact that populations are stratified in various ways. For example, we can estimate the total number of bacteria in a culture, but each cell is in a particular phase of its reproductive cycle. It is either replicating its DNA in preparation for splitting, or it is preparing for replication or it has just completed replication. These three phases of cell life can be further broken down, etc., but estimating the numbers of cells in each of these three phases is quite difficult. Similarly, we could estimate the total human population on earth or we could describe its structure, say stratified by age groups or by genetic traits such as gender, blood type, race, etc.

A further complication is that population growth is eventually limited by some resource, usually one from among many essential nutrients. When a population is far from its limits of growth, it can grow geometrically. However, when nearing its limits, the population size can fluctuate, even chaotically.

Our discussion of population numbers illustrates four methods that have been used successfully in studying them: First, we consider total population size when growth is unlimited. Next, we study the age structure of an unlimited population. Third, we consider total population size when growth is limited, and finally, we consider age structure in a population that is near its environment's carrying capacity. The chapter ends with a presentation of some management issues related to populations.

1.1 Geometric Population Growth

In this section, we will study the growth of a bacterial culture and how its growth rate can be estimated from experimental data. Then we consider cell doubling times.

1.1.1 GROWTH OF BACTERIAL CULTURES

Large batches of bacteria are important for many scientific and industrial projects. A typical procedure is to inoculate a jar containing growth media with a sample of cells taken from storage. The inoculum might contain 1.0 $\times 10^8$ cells/ml (ml denotes 1 milliliter). The inoculated mixture is then placed in an incubator and shaken for approximately 8 hours. After this time, there are approximately 1.0×10^{10} cells/ml. The batch culture can be sampled at regular time intervals, for example by drawing a sample of 1 ml and measuring its optical density. In this way, the concentration of cells in the growth chamber can be monitored. Typical data are presented in Table 1.1.

It is interesting to derive a mathematical model to "explain" these data. In particular, we would like to give some simple description of the population's growth that could perhaps be used to characterize the cell strain.

Let B_n denote the cell numbers observed at the nth sampling time: $B_0 =$ the initial cell concentration, $B_1 = 1.9 \times 10^8$, etc. We expect that during the growth phase the cell number at one time will be some multiple of the previous measurement and that this multiple will be constant over several

TABLE 1.1. Sampling Data for a Population of Salmonella Typhimurium at Hourly Intervals

Sample Time (hours)	Observed Density (cells/ml)
1	1.9×10^8
2	3.6×10^8
3	6.9×10^8
4	1.3×10^9
5	2.5×10^9
6	4.7×10^9
7	8.5×10^9
8	1.4×10^{10}

sampling times. In this hope, we write the equation

$$B_{n+1} = r\, B_n. \tag{1.1.1}$$

The constant r is called the *growth rate*, and it is this number that we will attempt to determine from the observations. If the cells divide every hour and our sampling is every hour, then we should observe that $r = 2$, and we say that the cell's *doubling time* is 1 hour.

In order to estimate r from the data, we use a statistical method called the *method of least-squares estimation*. This is described in the next section.

1.1.2   Least Squares Estimation of the Growth Rate

Suppose that data are observed, say $(x_1, y_1), \ldots, (x_N, y_N)$ and that a theory predicts that these data are linearly related, say

$$y = a\,x + b.$$

The parameters a and b should be chosen so that this relation "best fits" the data, and the least-squares method gives one way to do this.

First, we introduce a measure of how far the data deviate from a straight line. Let

$$L(a,b) = \sum_{i=1}^{N} (y_i - a\,x_i - b)^2.$$

The parameters a and b are chosen to minimize this quantity. If a and b do give a minimum, then

$$\frac{\partial L}{\partial a} = 0 \ \text{ and } \ \frac{\partial L}{\partial b} = 0.$$

So it is from among the solutions of these two equations that we seek a and b. These two equations can be written as

$$\begin{aligned}
a <x^2> \ + \ b <x> \ &= \ <xy> \\
a <x> \ + \ b\,N \ &= \ <y>
\end{aligned}$$

where

$$< x > = \sum_{i=1}^{N} x_i, \quad < y > = \sum_{i=1}^{N} y_i$$

and

$$< x^2 > = \sum_{i=1}^{N} x_i^2, \quad < xy > = \sum_{i=1}^{N} x_i \, y_i.$$

The solutions of these equations are

$$a = \frac{N < xy > - < x >< y >}{N < x^2 > - < x >^2}, \quad b = \frac{N < x^2 >< y > - < x >< xy >}{N < x^2 > - < x >^2}.$$

These constants are then used in the straight line formula to give the least-squares approximation.

This method can be used to estimate the bacterial growth rate r, but not directly. It only works if there is a linear relation between the data and the sampling times. Therefore, we next investigate the relation between B_n and n.

The model (1.1.1) can be solved for B_n. Starting with an arbitrary time, say n, we successively substitute backwards using the equation, and we get that

$$B_n = r \, B_{n-1} = r(r B_{n-2}) = \cdots = r^n B_0.$$

That is,

$$B_n = r^n B_0 \tag{1.1.2}$$

This is a convenient form for the solution of the model, and it shows that the number of cells at any time (n) depends only on n, r, and B_0. This formula also shows that the population grows geometrically with *common ratio r*.

It is apparent from the solution that B_n and n are not linearly related. However, if we take logarithms of the solution, we get

$$\log B_n = n \log r + \log B_0$$

where $\log r$ denotes the natural logarithm (base e) of r. Thus, the theory predicts that there is a linear relation between $\log B_n$ and n. Therefore, $x_1 = 1$, $y_1 = \log 1.9$, $x_2 = 2$, $y_2 = \log 3.6$, etc., from Table 1.1. The method of least squares gives the results in numbers a and b where a is an estimate of $\log r$. In this case $\log r = 0.642$, or $r = 1.9$. Compare the predicted solution with the data in Table 1.1.

1.1.3 GROWTH OF HUMAN POPULATIONS

These methods give remarkably good predictions of Sweden's population numbers for nearly a century (the percent error does not exceed 10%!) {see Ex. 1.1}. Similar calculations for Wales (1860–1960) are good to 1920, but lead to errors of more than 25% thereafter. The model is acceptable for some purposes over certain phases of growth, but it must eventually become invalid as a population reaches its limits of growth. Causes of this might lie in population size-dependent changes in the physical or biological environment, or in the age structure of the population.

In 1760, L. Euler suggested that populations grow geometrically, but as a result of later work by Malthus (1798) equation (1.1.1) is now called a *Malthusian model*. In the years following 1800, data were collected and analyzed to test such theories, and like the examples, populations were observed to grow geometrically during certain phases. We will account for the limits of growth later.

1.1.4 INFINITESIMAL SAMPLING INTERVALS AND DOUBLING TIMES

Bacteria have discrete generations, so when they are synchronized, they can be counted at fixed time intervals that are related to their biology. We did not do this in our earlier calculations, where we simply measured the total population every hour. However, human reproduction is not synchronized across the population by available nutrients, climate cues, etc., so there is no obvious choice for sampling intervals.

This problem can be avoided in part by studying infinitesimal sampling intervals. Let $P(t)$ denote the population size at time t, and suppose that the change observed over a short time interval, say of length h, is proportional to the population size. Since percent change of the population is small if the sampling interval h is small, we write $r = 1 + h\, b$: Then $P(t + h) = r\, P(t)$, or

$$P(t + h) - P(t) = h\, bP(t).$$

The number b is called the *net birth rate* or *intrinsic growth rate*. We view $P(t)$ as being a smooth function of t. Then, dividing by h and passing to the limit $h = 0$ gives the differential equation

$$\frac{dP}{dt} = b\, P \tag{1.1.3}$$

which we must solve for the population size $P(t)$. This is a differential equation version for overlapping generations of Malthus's model for discrete generations. Note that no assumption is made about synchrony of the population in this derivation, only about its instantaneous changes.

Equation (1.1.3) can be solved by the method of separation of variables. Dividing both sides of the equation by P and multiplying by dt gives

$$dP/P = b\, dt.$$

Integrating this equation from $t = 0$ to $t = T$ [thus, the left side from $P = P(0)$ to $P = P(T)$], we have

$$\log P(T) - \log P(0) = b\, T.$$

Equivalently,

$$P(T) = P(0)e^{bT}.$$

So, the population grows exponentially, which is the continuous time analog of geometric growth in synchronized populations.

The model of bacterial growth (1.1.1) is one based on population size at distinct time steps, $n = 0, 1, \ldots$, and the result is referred to as being a difference equation. There are many advantages in converting, when possible, a difference equation to one based on continuous time, as we have done here. In fact, calculus was introduced in large part to facilitate solving difference equations, and it often enables us to calculate solutions in a convenient form and to analyze solutions more efficiently than is possible for difference equations.

The solution of the discrete-time model, $B_n = r^n B_0$, and the solution of the overlapping generation model, $P(t) = P(0)e^{bt}$, are easy to connect: If we sample $P(t)$ at times nh where h is the length of the sampling interval, the resulting numbers should be related to the sequence B_n. Because of this, we set $P(nh) = B_n$, then $r^n = e^{bnh}$. Equivalently, $b = (1/h)\log r$. In the bacterial sampling data in Table 1.1, $h = 1.0$ hours.

This observation enables us to derive the cell doubling time from the data presented at the start of this section. We ask, what time T is needed so that $P(T) = 2P(0)$? Thus, $e^{bT} = 2.0$ or

$$T = \log 2/b = \log 2/\log r.$$

Since $r = 1.9$, we have that the doubling time is $T = 1.07$ hours, which is different from the sampling time interval, but close to it.

1.2 Geometric Growth in a Population Stratified by Age

We begin with a very old story that describes age structure in a synchronized population. The ideas are later generalized to study human populations that have synchronized generations and that have overlapping generations.

1.2.1 FIBONACCI'S RABBIT POPULATION

Age structure of a population is more difficult to deal with than total population size, but the following example, Fibonacci's model, introduces the basic ideas of age structure in a simple way. Fibonacci proposed (in 1202!) a model for population growth based on an imaginary rabbit population. We start with one pair of rabbits (one female and one male) that matures to reproductive age, say N days old. At that time they produce a new pair, one female and one male. The original pair will survive to the next reproductive time (N days later) and again produce a pair. Each pair of rabbits will reproduce twice, at intervals separated by N days, and at each reproduction the new pair will go on in a similar fashion. All of the reproduction is synchronized and each pair reproduces exactly twice.

Fibonacci's population can be modeled using the numbers
$R_n =$ the number of pairs that are born at the nth time.
Then the first pair appears at $n = 0$ and bears one pair at $n = 1$:

$$R_0 = 1$$
$$R_1 = 1$$

and for all later times

$$R_n = R_{n-1} + R_{n-2} \quad \text{for} \quad n = 2, 3, 4, \ldots \tag{1.2.1}$$

so $R_2 = R_1 + R_0 = 2, R_3 = R_2 + R_1 = 2 + 1 = 3$, etc. The fact that we are accounting for the age structure, namely the fact that each pair reproduces at two separate ages N and $2N$ days old, is reflected in the two-step difference equation (1.2.1) for the sequence of population sizes R_n where the number of births now depends on both the population sizes N and $2N$ days ago.

The analysis of this iteration has intrigued mathematicians for centuries: We could continue as earlier to evaluate the entire *Fibonacci sequence*, 1,1,2,3,5,8,13, ..., where each term is the sum of the preceding two, but this quickly becomes pointless.

Fortunately, it is possible to find a convenient solution of this problem. Experience with Malthus's model suggests that we look for the term R_n as a power of some common ratio [see **2**]:

$$R_n = r^n.$$

Substituting this into the equation, we see that r must satisfy the equation

$$r^2 - r - 1 = 0$$

which has two solutions

$$r = \frac{1 \pm \sqrt{5}}{2}.$$

It follows that the terms in the sequence are given by the formula

$$R_n = A\, r_1^n + B\, r_2^n$$

where

$$r_1 = \frac{1 + \sqrt{5}}{2}, \quad r_2 = \frac{1 - \sqrt{5}}{2}$$

$$A = \frac{1 + \sqrt{5}}{2\sqrt{5}}, \quad B = \frac{1 - \sqrt{5}}{2\sqrt{5}}.$$

The constants A and B are determined from the first two terms of the population sequence: $R_0 = 1$ and $R_1 = 1$. Remarkably, this works!

Two surprising results of this formula are:

1. Although complicated, this expression for R_n always gives an integer!

2. The ratio $R_n/R_{n-1} \to (1 + \sqrt{5})/2 = 1.618\ldots$ as n increases.

The second point shows that Fibonacci's sequence is a sequence of integers that grows (almost) geometrically.

Although Fibonacci's model is artificial, it nicely illustrates important methods used to study more realistic age-structured problems. Exercises 1.2 and 1.12 illustrate other features and extensions of this model.

1.2.2 EULER'S RENEWAL EQUATIONS

Fibonacci's model suggests how we could describe real populations. In fact, Euler described the age structure of human populations in 1760. Now, we consider a population that we count at specific census intervals, but we only keep track of the newborn females. Let B_n denote the number of females born during the nth census period.

The population is divided into age classes, each a census period long. Those in the kth age class are survivors of those born k periods earlier. Then those who reach census age k can contribute to births in it. B_{n-k} denotes the number of females born in census $n - k$, so the survivors of them at time n have (census) age k. Their chronological age is k times the census interval which is usually 5 or 10 years. We denote by λ_k the proportion of those born k censuses ago who survived. Thus, λ_k is the probability of a newborn surviving from birth to the kth census. We denote by b_k the fertility of those in their k^{th} census interval. Therefore, the individuals born k censuses ago are expected to produce $b_k \lambda_k B_{n-k}$ daughters during the kth census. Finally, there might be some births in the nth census interval from those who were present when we started counting everything, and we lump all of these into one number h_n.

Adding up all of these numbers, we get the number of births in the nth census interval to be

$$B_n = h_n + b_1\lambda_1 B_{n-1} + b_2\lambda_2 B_{n-2} + + \ldots + b_n\lambda_n B_0. \qquad (1.2.2)$$

This equation is referred to as the *renewal equation*. In Fibonacci's case, $\lambda_j = 1$ for all j, and $b_1 = b_2 = 1$ and $b_j = 0$ for $j \geq 3$.

The numbers $\{\lambda_k\}$ have been tabulated for many human populations, and the results are summarized in what is called a *life table*. Birth rate data for these populations give the fertilities $\{b_k\}$. A wealth of data and interesting examples are given in the reference book by Keyfitz and Flieger [1].

There are various ways of extracting useful information from the renewal equation. Fibonacci's model demonstrates the usual method, and we take the same point of view toward solving (1.2.2). Here the data for the life table and the fertilities are assumed to be known, say with fertility zero for large ages, $b_k = 0$ for $k > M$, so $h_n = 0$ for $n > M$ as well.

For example, a census interval might be 5 years, and since female fertility stops by age 55 (approximately), $M = 11$.

Let us suppose that $B_n \sim r^n$. Therefore, for $n > M$,

$$r^n = b_1 \lambda_1 r^{n-1} + \ldots + b_M \lambda_M r^{n-M}$$

or equivalently (multiplying by r^M)

$$r^M = b_1 \lambda_1 r^{M-1} + \ldots + b_M \lambda_M.$$

This is an Mth order polynomial for r. It is similar to the second order polynomial for r that we derived for Fibonacci's model. There will be M roots for r, say $r_1, \ldots, r_M$, and the solution for B_n will have the form

$$B_n = A_1 r_1^n + \ldots + A_M r_M^n \quad \text{for} \quad n = 1, 2 \ldots,$$

for some constants $A_1, A_2, \ldots, A_M$. This formula generalizes the one we found for R_n in Fibonacci's rabbit population [see **2**].

The following result is very important. Although we do not prove it here, its validity is quite plausible. First, we define

$$p = \sum_{k=0}^{M} b_k \lambda_k.$$

This is the expected number of female offspring that each newborn will produce in her entire life. We state the results as a theorem

Renewal Theorem: Let the fertilities $b_0, \ldots, b_M$, and the life table $\lambda_0, \ldots, \lambda_M$, be given, and let p be the expected number of daughters each newborn will bear. Then

1. If $p < 1, B_n \to 0$ as $n \to \infty$. That is, if each newborn less than replaces herself over her lifetime, the population will die out.

2. If $p \geq 1$ and if there is a unique *positive* root of the characteristic equation

$$r^M - b_1 \lambda_1 r^{M-1} - \ldots - b_M \lambda_M = 0 \qquad (1.2.3)$$

for r, say r^*, then all other roots satisfy $\mid r \mid < r^*$, and

$$\lim_{t \to \infty} r^{*-n} B_n = C$$

where C is a constant.

The value $p = 1$ is a threshold value for the population's birth and death rates. If each newborn will more than replace herself ($p > 1$), then the number of newborns grows geometrically since

$$B_n \sim C \, r^{*n}$$

for large values of n. The constant C can be determined using a method that is not described here [see **2**], but in any case, the values of C and r^* can be

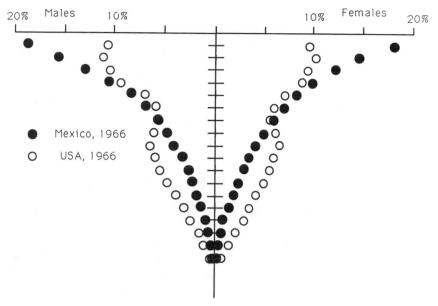

FIGURE 1.1. Age pyramid.

estimated from population data using the least squares estimation method as in Section 1.1.2 {Ex. 1.11}.

The technical condition that there be a unique dominant root of 1.2.3 is usually satisfied, but it is needed to rule out cases where fertility is focused in just a few age groups, like in insect populations. This is discussed in Section 1.4.

The renewal equation is widely used for predicting population age structures, and once the birth rates $\{B_n\}$ are known, the entire population can be reconstructed since the number of individuals expected in the nth census who were born k intervals before now is $B_{n-k}\lambda_k$. Often this distribution among the age groups is plotted as a histogram, as shown in Figure 1.1.

1.2.3* AGE STRUCTURE IN HUMAN POPULATIONS

A renewal equation can be derived in the case of infinitesimal census intervals. Let $B(t)$ denote the number of births at time t, let $b(a)$ be the fertility of a female of age a, and let $\lambda(a)$ denote the probability of a newborn surviving to age a. Then the number of females of age a at time t is

$$\lambda(a)B(t-a)$$

and the number of offspring they produce in a short interval, say of length da, is

$$\lambda(a)b(a)B(t-a)da.$$

Adding these up and adding in the contributions from the initial population, we have the *renewal equation*

$$B(t) = h(t) + \int_0^t b(a)\lambda(a)B(t-a)da \qquad (1.2.4)$$

This integral equation is to be solved for $B(t)$. While the equation was easy to derive, its solution is not so easy to find. Fortunately, there is a method, called the *Laplace transform method* [3] that shows how to find $B(t)$ {see Ex. 1.13}.

The answer has the form

$$B(t) = A\,e^{r*t} + \quad \text{smaller terms.} \qquad (1.2.5)$$

As we have seen in the previous cases, the birth rate B winds up growing exponentially.

Laplace's method does for this equation what we did for Fibonacci's equation by setting $R_n = r^n$. Instead of guessing that the solution is a geometric progression, we guess here that it is an exponential function. An equation for r^* can be found by setting $B(t) = e^{rt}$ and substituting in the renewal equation. When t is large enough so that $h(t) = 0$, then the result is

$$1 = \int_0^\infty e^{-ra}\lambda(a)\,b(a)\,da.$$

A solution of this equation is $r = r^*$. Although these calculations fall mostly outside the scope of this text, they show two things important to us here:

1. It is possible to model a population's age structure using infinitesimal sampling intervals, and the resulting model can be solved using calculus.

2. The births and so the total population behave like Malthus's model predicts: In fact, from Equation (1.2.5) the total population is

$$\int_0^t \lambda(a)B(t-a)da \approx \int_0^t A\,e^{r*(t-a)}\lambda(a)\,da \approx A\,e^{r*t}\int_0^T \lambda(a)\,e^{-r*a}da$$

where "$\sim$" means "=" except for some small terms and T is the largest possible age of survival. Thus, the total population behaves like a Malthusian population, even when we account for its age structure.

1.3   The Limits of Growth

Malthus's model proposes a simple relationship between two successive measurements of population size, but careful experiments using bacteria and insects and careful observations of human populations, some dating back to the middle of the last century, suggest that whereas this is often valid during a certain phase of a population's growth, more complicated relationships are usually needed. Crowding of a population can suppress reproduction in a variety of ways: increased stress placed on individuals or reduced nutrition can reduce fertility, and depletion of essential nutrients can cause more deaths. Therefore, as the population grows, its growth rate should be expected eventually to decrease. This happens even in the data in Table 1.1 where the predicted sizes $(1.9)^n$ and the observed sizes diverge at $n = 7, 8$.

A reproduction rule more general than Malthus's has the form

$$P_{n+1} = R(P_n)P_n \tag{1.3.1}$$

where $R(P)$ is the *intrinsic growth rate* when the population is of size P. This model might describe the population over a wider range, but the problem of estimating $R(P)$ from data must be solved.

1.3.1 VERHULST'S MODEL

Consider a strain of bacteria that are *histidine auxotrophs*; that is, they cannot produce their own histidine, an amino acid needed to construct proteins and make possible cell reproduction. When these bacteria are cultured in growth media containing sufficient histidine, they double in size and divide every 40 minutes. Let us begin with a known number of cells, say B_0, at time zero and monitor the population size at successive division times. Let $B_1 =$ number of cells after 40 minutes, $B_2 =$ number of cells after 80 minutes, etc. The simple formula

$$B_{n+1} = 2\, B_n$$

describes the population measurements when there is adequate histidine and other necessary nutrients and when the doubling time is 40 minutes. In this case, $R(B) = 2$.

When the number of cells becomes large, competition for the limited amount of histidine ensues, and the bacteria get an inadequate supply to sustain division every 40 minutes. Thus, observations every 40 minutes no longer are synchronized with the division cycle.

To describe the population despite the increased doubling time, we no longer count single identifiable cells but describe only the total cell mass present in the growth chamber at the end of each 40 minute interval. We suppose that if a newborn daughter cell has mass M, after maturation it has mass $2M$ and after splitting there are two daughters, each having mass M. The total mass of cells after n intervals, which we denote by C_n, equals $B_n M$ in the optimal case, and as long as C_n is not large

$$C_{n+1} = 2\, C_n.$$

However, when the population is large, it less than reproduces itself each interval. We could describe this by setting

$$C_{n+1} = \frac{2}{1 + \frac{C_n}{K}} C_n. \tag{1.3.2}$$

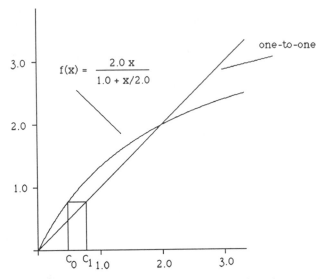

FIGURE 1.2. Reproduction curve for limited environments.

Studies of histidine uptake by growing cells recommend this form where K, called the *saturation constant*, is characteristic of the cell strain and the growth media. When $C = K$, the reproduction is only one half its maximum. In this model, the larger the cell mass becomes, the smaller will be the increase in total cell mass every 40 minutes.

A model similar to this one was derived by Verhulst in 1848 as a result of studies of certain human populations [1]. For this reason, Equation (1.3.1) is referred to here as being *Verhulst's model*. It has also appeared in the fishery literature where it is called the *Beverton–Holt* model [4].

This model is not as easy to solve as the earlier one was, but we can find its solution in a number of interesting ways. For example, we can plot the solutions by plotting the points (C_n, C_{n+1}) on coordinate axes as shown in Figure 1.2.

A one-to-one reference line is also plotted for convenience. This plot, called the *reproduction curve*, often can be used to determine the cell population's dynamics. Given an initial cell concentration, C_0, the concentration after 1 hour, C_1, is determined from the graph. This value is reflected in the one-to-one reference line as shown in Figure 1.2.

The process can be repeated, as in Figure 1.3. This shows that if $C_0 < K$, then C_n increases up toward K in successive intervals. The graphical method described here is called *cobwebbing*, or Picard's method; it provides an easy way to sketch population dynamics.

On the other hand, it is actually possible to derive a closed form solution to the model (1.3.2). We can transform the equation into one where successive back substitutions can be easily carried out. In this case, we define new

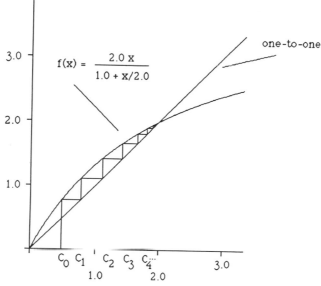

FIGURE 1.3. Geometric iteration.

variables $R_0, R_1, \ldots$, by setting

$$R_n = 1/C_n.$$

Then the sequence $\{R_n\}$ satisfies a linear relationship

$$R_{n+1} = R_n/2 + (1/2K)$$

Successive back substitutions show that

$$
\begin{aligned}
R_{n+1} &= R_n/2 + (1/2K) \\
&= R_{n-1}/2^2 + (1/4K) + (1/2K) \\
&= (1/2)^{n+1} R_0 + (1/2K)\{1 + \ldots + (1/2)^n\}.
\end{aligned}
$$

The last term here enclosed in braces { } is a geometric progression, and it can be evaluated directly using the formula

$$1 + \ldots + \left(\frac{1}{2}\right)^n = \frac{1 - \left(\frac{1}{2}\right)^{n+1}}{1 - \frac{1}{2}}.$$

Therefore, $R_{n+1} \to 1/K$ as $n \to \infty$, or equivalently, $C_n \to K$. K is apparently the media's *carrying capacity* for this strain of bacteria.

Since the equation for the reciprocal masses R_n is linear, we can use the least-squares method to estimate the carrying capacity K from experimental data.

Unfortunately, there are many other choices possible for $R(P)$, and some of them have remarkable properties.

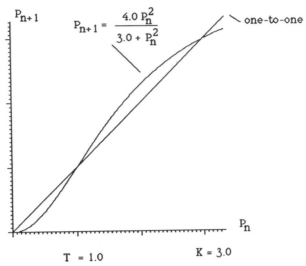

FIGURE 1.4. Predator satiation threshold.

1.3.2   PREDATOR SATIATION

In ecological systems, say where there are prey and predators, or in the human immune system, which responds to a bacterial infection with predatory phage cells, there is a threshold size of their numbers below which the prey or bacteria are completely eliminated. This can be accounted for by setting

$$R(P) = \frac{rP}{1 + \left(\frac{P}{K}\right)^2}$$

The resulting model is

$$P_{n+1} = \left(\frac{rP_n^2}{1 + \left(\frac{P_n}{K}\right)^2}\right).$$

Now, however, we cannot solve this equation in closed form using the back substitution method. In this case, we rely on the plotting, or cobwebbing, method to sketch solutions for the various choices of r and K, but we do not attempt to estimate these parameters. The reproduction curve is drawn in Figure 1.4.

Critical population sizes are where $R(P) = 1$. These occur when

$$P = 0 \quad \text{and} \quad P = K\left(\frac{rK}{2} \pm \sqrt{\left(\frac{rK}{2}\right)^2 - 1}\right).$$

Let us denote the middle of these three roots by T, and the larger one by K^*, as shown in Figure 1.4. A population starting below T will less than reproduce itself, so it dies out. Above this, the population will establish itself at the stable carrying capacity, $P = K^*$.

The interval $0 < P < T$ is a *pit of extinction* since once a population is forced into it, for example by a significant change in its environment, there is no return.

1.3.3 CHAOS

As simple as the model (1.3.1) appears to be, there lie nearby very complicated issues. We have seen cases where we could solve the equation by successive back substitution and where at least we could sketch solutions using the cobwebbing method to determine how the solutions behave. However, even the plotting method might not work! We illustrate this remarkable fact in this section.

It happens that reproduction can actually decrease as population sizes become large and crowding occurs. For example, adult guppies will feed on their young so the offspring of an extremely large adult population will face little chance of survival. Although populations of intermediate size will more than reproduce themselves, large ones may not.

A simple model of this is given by Equation (1.3.1) with

$$R(P) = r \exp(-P/K)$$

where r is the maximum reproduction rate (when the population is small) and K is the population size at which the reproduction rate is approximately half its maximum. The model was introduced by Ricker [5] in 1954 to study fish populations, but other models have been studied as well. The model is

$$P_{n+1} = r \, e^{-P_n/K} P_n. \qquad (1.3.3)$$

This model is one of the first to produce "chaos," a term introduced in 1975 [see 6] to describe highly unpredictable dynamics of otherwise simple looking systems.

If $r < 1$, then the population will always less than replace itself and so die out. However, if r is greater than 1, a small population will more than replace itself, and the equilibrium value $P^* = K \log r$ is a likely result of iteration. This might or might not be the case depending on the size of r. If $1 < r < r^*$, where

$$r^* = e^{-\frac{P^*}{K}} \left(1 - \frac{P^*}{K} \right) = -1$$

then the iterates will approach $P^* r^*$ is the value of r for which

$$\left(\frac{d(R(P)P)}{dP} \right) = -1.$$

However, for $r > r^*$ the solutions do other things, as indicated in Table 1.2.

When $r = 10.0$, the population numbers settle to a simple oscillation between two numbers 36706 and 9346. However, when $r = 20.0$, the population

TABLE 1.2. Population Data Generated by Ricker's Model when $K = 10000$ and $P_0 = 5000$, for $r = 20.0$ and for $r = 10.0$

n	$P_n(r = 20.0)$	$P_n(r = 10.0)$
0	5000	5000
1	60653	30326
2	2817	14614
3	42506	33892
4	12119	11434
5	72140	36444
6	1062	9525
7	19103	36745
8	56558	9319
9	3956	36699
10	53268	9351
11	5177	36707
12	61701	9345
13	2580	36706
14	39871	9346
15	14795	36706
16	67391	9346
17	1595	36706
18	27202	9346
19	35830	36706
20	19916	9346

numbers seem to be random. Of course, they are not random since there is a complete correlation between P_{n+1} and $R(P_n)P_n$. A more sophisticated approach was introduced in 1975 [see **7**] to describe the distribution of the iterates of this model for various values of r.

A computer can be used to describe the solutions when things get this complicated. To do this, we use the following program: First, since the derivative of $R(P)P$ equals zero when $P = K$, the maximum value of $R(P)P$ occurs when $P = K$, so the range of this reproduction function is $0 \leq P \leq rK/e$. We next normalize the variables by setting $Q = eP/rK$, so the range of Q will be $0 \leq Q \leq 1$. Substituting for P, we get the model

$$Q_{n+1} = r\, Q_n\, e^{-rQ_n/e}.$$

Next, we split the interval $0 \leq Q \leq 1$ into many equal subintervals. We select an initial point and iterate it many times, recording each time an iterate hits one of the subintervals. We then list the results as a histogram over these subintervals

Let us repeat the experiments described in Table 1.2. First, we convert the data in Table 1.2 from P variables to Q: Next, we partition the interval $0 \leq Q \leq 1$ into 10 equal subintervals, each of length 0.10. Then we create a histogram for each of these sets of data as shown in Table 1.4.

The data in Table 1.2 describe 20 iterations of the reproduction function for each of the two values: $r = 20.0$ and $r = 10.0$. The two histograms in Table 1.4 depict the results of these iterations. The number of $*$'s in each histogram add up to 20, the total number of iterations. In the case $r = 20.0$, the iterates are spread throughout the intervals, although roughly one half of them are in the first interval. In the case $r = 10.0$, there are a few iterates outside the two cells containing 0.25 and 0.95, but most of the iterates are in those two cells, equal numbers in each. The few outside of them describe transients as the process settles down. By carrying out this iteration and plotting the histograms, we can get a picture of the iteration's dynamics, even though the geometrical method of cobwebbing tells us little in the case of $r = 20.0$ because the cobweb gets too dense.

The more organized the histograms, the more regular is the behavior of the iterations. We can quantify how spread out the histograms are by calculating their *entropy*.

Suppose that we end up with a histogram having iterates distributed among the M subintervals with frequencies $f_1, f_2, \ldots, f_M$. We could calculate various statistics of this distribution (e.g., mean, variance, kurtosis, etc.). However, we will only try to quantify how spread out is the distribution, which can be done using its entropy. The *entropy* is defined by the number

$$H(f_1, \ldots, f_M) = -\frac{1}{\log M} \sum_{j=1}^{M} f_j \log\, f_j$$

where we define $f_j \log f_j = 0$ if $f_j = 0$. H has the following interesting properties:

TABLE 1.3. The Data in Table 1.2 Converted to the Q Variable by scaling: $Q = eP/rK$

n	$Q_n(r = 20.0)$	$Q_n(r = 10.0)$
0	0.0680	0.1359
1	0.8244	0.8243
2	0.0383	0.3972
3	0.5777	0.9213
4	0.1647	0.3108
5	0.9805	0.0990
6	0.0144	0.2589
7	0.2596	0.9988
8	0.7687	0.2533
9	0.0538	0.9976
10	0.7240	0.2542
11	0.0704	0.9978
12	0.8386	0.2540
13	0.0351	0.9978
14	0.5419	0.2540
15	0.2011	0.9978
16	0.9159	0.2540
17	0.0217	0.9978
18	0.3697	0.2540
19	0.4870	0.9978
20	0.2707	0.2540

TABLE 1.4. Histograms for Data in Table 1.3

Q values	Frequency,	$\#(r = 20)$	Frequency,	$\#(r = 10)$
$[0.0, 0.1)$	0.30	******	0.05	*
$[0.1, 0.2)$	0.05	*		
$[0.2, 0.3)$	0.15	***	0.40	********
$[0.3, 0.4)$	0.05	*	0.10	**
$[0.4, 0.5)$	0.05	*		
$[0.5, 0.6)$	0.10	**		
$[0.6, 0.7)$	0.00			
$[0.7, 0.8)$	0.10	**		
$[0.8, 0.9)$	0.10	**	0.05	*
$[0.9, 1.0]$	0.10	**	0.40	********

TABLE 1.5. Entropy of the Histograms in Table 1.4.

r	Entropy
20.0	0.6729
10.0	0.4216

1. $H(f_1, \ldots, f_M)$ is a smooth function of its arguments for which each $f_j \geq 0$ and $\sum f_j = 1.0$.

2. $0 \leq H(f_1, \ldots, f_M) \leq 1.0$ for any distribution f as in 1.

3. If all data are in one cell, say $f_J = 1$, then $H = 0.0$. This is the only case when $H = 0.0$.

4. If all iterations are uniformly distributed (i.e. $f_j = 1/M$) then $H = 1.0$, its maximum value. In fact, $H < 1.0$ for all other distributions.

Therefore, the smaller H is, the more organized is the histogram; i.e., the fewer are the cells that are hit by the iteration. When $H = 1.0$, then the behavior is chaotic since all cells are hit repeatedly by the iteration.

The entropy of the two histograms in Table 1.4 are shown in Table 1.5. After many more than 20 iterations, the transients in the second case ($r = 10.0$) become less important, and we would have an entropy (approximately) equal to $\log 2/\log 20 = 0.2313$. If we drop the first five iterations in Table 1.2 to suppress transients, all future iterates lie in the two cells containing 0.25 and 0.95, and the entropy will be exactly 0.2313!

The two histograms in Table 1.4 were constructed using a hand calculator. Using the random number generator on a calculator 20 times gives a histogram having entropy 0.7136. It is clear that taking as few iterations as we have done here does not give a clear picture of the dynamics, but it suggests what is happening, and it points the way to a good use of a computer or an extended session with a hand calculator {Ex. 1.3}.

The results of a computer simulation are described in Figure 1.5. Plotted on the horizontal axis are the values of r, ranging from 0.0 to 25.0. In the bottom graph we plot the cells of the Q interval $0 \leq Q \leq 1$, of which we have created 1000. We ignore the first 50 of 10,000 iterations, and create a histogram for each value of r. Rather than plotting the histogram in three dimensions, we look straight down on it and plot a point if a cell is occupied. For the same value of r, we plot in the top figure the entropy of the histogram. We see that for $r < r^* \sim 8$ there is a single occupied cell, and the iterates tend to a constant population size. For $8 < r < 13$, all iterates eventually oscillate between two sizes, a large one and a small one. This was illustrated in Table 1.4. Things get more complicated beyond $r = 13.0$. The entropy successively increases, for some values of r becoming almost 1.0, but surprisingly it drops to very low values for some other r values. Values where H is large are values for which the dynamics are chaotic {Exs. 1.4, 1.5}.

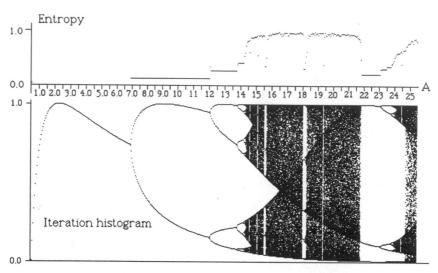

FIGURE 1.5. Histogram for Ricker's model.

1.3.4   Infinitesimal Sampling Intervals in a Limiting Environment

When the reproduction rate changes with population size, it may be impossible to determine a natural sampling time for experiments or to observe the population at natural times. In many cases, we can benefit again by considering infinitesimal sampling times.

Recall Verhulst's model (1.3.1)

$$P_{n+1} = \frac{rP_n}{1 + \frac{P_n}{K}}.$$

If the sampling time is short and the population is not large, we may write $r = 1 + h$, and since $P_n \to P^* = (r-1)K = h\,K$, we write $P = h\,p$. Then

$$p_{n+1} - p_n = h\,p_n(1 - p_n/K)/(1 + hp_n/K).$$

If we expect to find a smooth function $p(t)$ for which $p_n = p(nh)$, then p must satisfy the differential equation that we obtain by dividing both sides by h and passing to the limit $h = 0$; namely,

$$dp/dt = p(1 - p/K).$$

This equation is known as the *logistic equation*, and it can be solved for $p(t)$ using the method of separation of variables and integration by partial fractions: Rearranging terms in the equation for $p(t)$ gives

$$dt = dp/p + dp/K(1 - p/K).$$

Therefore, integrating this formula gives

$$t = \log\{p(t)(K - p(0))/(K - p(t))p(0)\}$$

or, solving for $p(t)$, we get {Ex. 1.7}

$$p(t) = Kp(0)e^t/\{K + p(0)(e^t - 1)\}.$$

Although this looks like a complicated formula, it is quite useful. For example, we see that as $t \to \infty$, then $p(t) \to K$ if $p(0) > 0$.

Therefore, the infinitesimal sampling model of Verhulst's equation predicts the same kind of behavior as the discrete generation model. However, simple differential equations of the form $dp/dt = f(p)$ cannot have chaotic solutions, so there is no scaling of Ricker's model (1.3.3) that will lead to an infinitesimal sampling interval model having chaotic dynamics.

Another kind of model can account for changes in a limiting nutrient and at the same time for the population size. For example, consider a batch culture of bacteria, say a bottle of nutrient media inoculated with a colony of *Salmonella typhimurium*. Let $P(t)$ denote the concentration (mass/volume) of cells at time t, and let $N(t)$ denote the concentration of a limiting nutrient. The cells might be histidine auxotrophs and the limiting nutrient might be histidine.

We suppose that the population grows at a rate that is dependent on the nutrient concentration, say $b(N)$ where $b(0) = 0$. Thus,

$$dP/dt = b(N)P.$$

There is a maximal growth rate that is realized when nutrient is abundant (N large), so we write

$$b(N) = V\,N/(K + N)$$

where Y, V, and K are constants. Y is the *bacterial yield* per unit of nutrient taken up by a cell, V is the *uptake velocity*, and K is the *saturation constant*. When the nutrient concentration is K, then the growth rate b is $YV/2$, half the possible maximum. The term

$$V\,N/(K + N)Y$$

is the amount of nutrient taken up per cell, and the total change in the nutrient concentration is

$$\frac{dN}{dt} = -\frac{V\,N\,P}{K + N} \cdot \frac{1}{Y}$$

Combining these equations leads to the model

$$\frac{dP}{dt} = \frac{V\,N\,P}{K + N}$$

$$\frac{dN}{dt} = -\frac{1}{Y}\frac{V\,N\,P}{K + N}.$$

(1.3.4)

These equations, which were introduced by *Jacob* and *Monod*, describe simultaneously cell growth and nutrient depletion.

This model is more complicated than our earlier ones since there are now two differential equations to be solved simultaneously. That can be done, but there is a short cut calculation that simplifies the problem: Consider the ratio of the two equations:

$$dP = -Y \, dN.$$

Therefore, we see that the quantity

$$P + Y N = \quad \text{constant.}$$

This formula shows that the total nutrient is conserved in the model that we derived when both the consumed nutrient (P/Y) and the unused nutrient (N) are taken into account. Integrating this equation gives the formula

$$P(t) - P(0) = Y(N(0) - N(t)).$$

Thus, a change in the bacterial population is proportional to the amount of nutrient used; on the other hand, an increment of nutrient used results in an increment of Y in the cell mass. This formula can be substituted in the first equation in (1.3.4), and the resulting equation for P alone can be solved using the methods described earlier {see Ex. 1.8}.

The constants Y, V, and K can be determined from experiments using the least-squares method of estimation. For example, the constant YV/K can be estimated by determining the doubling time when small amounts of N are made available. The maximum growth rate V can be estimated from the population when nutrient is abundant, and the saturation constant K can be estimated by titrating nutrient down from abundance to where the population's doubling time is half its maximum observed value.

1.4   Age Structure of Populations Near the Limits of Growth

Insects, such as cicadas, that have a many year life cycle remain as immature young for many years and as adults capable of reproducing the last. Adult cicadas reproduce in trees by laying fertilized eggs on branches. Their offspring drop to the ground and hatch as nymphs who enter the ground and attach to tree rootlets for nourishment. After a certain number of years, they change form. At the right time, they emerge from the ground, change to a flying form, and fly to the branches to reproduce. Then the reproduction cycle repeats. One interesting observation made of cicada populations is that short-lived ones (7-year lifespans or less) seem to appear in comparable numbers every year, while longer lived ones (say 13 years) appear only every 13 years. The cohorts are distinct from year to year, but somehow they become synchronized.

Some insight to this can be gained by considering an organism that has a 2-year life cycle where after 1 year, newborns become immature youths and

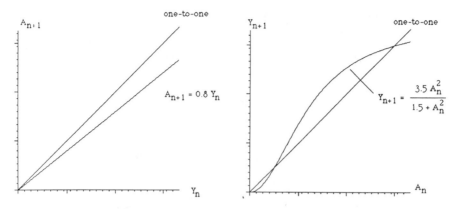

FIGURE 1.6. Reproduction curve for two age classes.

after 2 years mature adults. There are a variety of insect and fish species, pacific salmon among them, that have such life cycles.

Let Y_n denote the number of immature young in year n, and let A_n be the number of mature adults. The number of adults in year $n + 1$ will be some proportion of the young, namely those that survive to reproductive age:

$$A_{n+1} = \sigma \, Y_n \qquad (1.4.1)$$

where σ, called the *survival probability*, is the probability of survival of a youth to maturity. The number of young next year will depend on the number of adults this year. We write

$$Y_{n+1} = f(A_n) \qquad (1.4.2)$$

where f describes the reproduction relation between breeding adults and next year's young. If predators must be satisfied during reproduction periods, then f will have the form already studied in Section 1.3.3. (Figure 1.6) These relations can be plotted simultaneously, as shown in Figure 1.7

A modification of the cobwebbing method helps in determining the dynamics of such a structured population. This modification is based on the observation that in cobwebbing the key ingredients are the horizontal axis, the

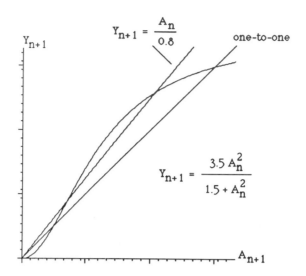

FIGURE 1.7. Combined reproduction curves.

one-to-one reference line, and the reproduction curve. The vertical axis plays no essential role in the procedure because we reflect in the one-to-one line. Therefore, we combine the two figures in Figure 1.6 on the same coordinate axes. This is shown in Figure 1.7

The iteration begins with an initial point (Y_1, A_1) and determines the next point (Y_2, A_2) as shown in Figure 1.8.

This procedure illustrates an interesting feature of such populations: There are three different kinds of behavior depending on the initial distribution of adults and juveniles. These initial regions are shown in Figure 1.9.

If (Y_0, A_0) lies in Region I, then (Y_n, A_n) approaches $(0,0)$ in successive years, and the population becomes extinct. Populations beginning in region III approach the point with coordinates (Y^*, A^*) and so equilibrate to a static state. Finally, populations that begin in either part of region II eventually alternate between the point $(Y^*, 0)$ and $(0, A^*)$. Such alternating behavior indicates that one of the year classes, or cohorts, becomes extinct while the other persists. In particular, adult breeding stock will appear only every other year. Thus, we see that three quite different results occur depending initially on only the population distribution among ages and their sizes.

Region I is referred to as the *extinction region*, Region III as the *balanced emergence* region, and Region II as the *synchronized emergence* region. Synchronized and balanced emergence regions are observed in insect and fish populations. Exercise 1.9 studies the cases of 7-, 13-, and 17-year cicadas.

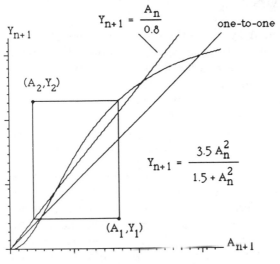

$$Y_{n+1} = \frac{A_n}{0.8}$$

one-to-one

Y_{n+1}

(A_2, Y_2)

$$Y_{n+1} = \frac{3.5\, A_n^2}{1.5 + A_n^2}$$

(A_1, Y_1)

A_{n+1}

FIGURE 1.8. First iteration.

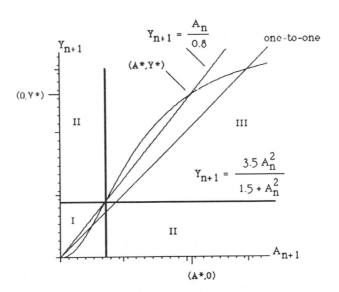

$$Y_{n+1} = \frac{A_n}{0.8}$$

one-to-one

Y_{n+1}

(A^*, Y^*)

$(0, Y^*)$

II   III

$$Y_{n+1} = \frac{3.5\, A_n^2}{1.5 + A_n^2}$$

I

II

A_{n+1}

$(A^*, 0)$

FIGURE 1.9. Regions of various behavior.

1.5 Harvesting

We produce food by harvesting crops and animals, and we produce new biotechnology products by harvesting microorganisms and byproducts of their metabolism. In this section, we see how harvesting can be described using the models in this chapter.

Suppose that we have a population whose dynamics are described by a reproduction relation of the form

$$P_{n+1} = f(P_n).$$

To fix ideas, we might consider the population to be one of fish, and the numbers P_n describe the fish population at the end of the nth annual season. Whatever the underlying biological system, we will consider one harvest each interval taken from among the new recruits to the population. For example, the population we are modeling might be the mature adult population, and $f(P)$ in model (1.3.1) denotes the number of new recruits to this population based on the adult population at the end of the previous interval. Therefore, we write

$$P_{n+1} = f(P_n) - h_n$$

where h_n is the harvest taken at the beginning of the $(n+1)^{st}$ interval, and P_{n+1} denotes the population at the end of this interval after harvesting.

Our first question is: What is the largest sustained yield that this population will produce? Let us denote the yield by Y. If the population is at equilibrium size P and steadily producing a yield Y, then

$$Y = f(P) - P.$$

The maximum of this function occurs where

$$\frac{df}{dP} - 1 = 0.$$

Therefore, a population P^* might produce a maximum sustained yield if $(df/dP)(P^*) = 1$. Let us suppose that $f(P) = PR(P)$.

As a harvesting policy, we might adjust the population size to reach P^*, and then it will maintain itself as we collect its yield $Y^* = (R(P^*) - 1)P^*$. Unfortunately, many populations that we deal with are not observable, such as wild fish populations. In those cases we must take a more sophisticated approach.

Two observables are the effort expended in harvesting and the yield that it produces. We make the following assumption that relates effort and yield: *Effort–Yield Relationship:* A unit effort produces a harvest of size $q\,P$ from a population of size P. q is the coefficient of catchability.

The effort needed to sustain yield Y in the equilibrium model is then found by adding the effort needed to reduce the population from $R(P)P$ to P one unit at a time. The effort-yield relationship leads to the formula

$$E = \frac{1}{q} \sum_{k=P}^{R(P)P} \frac{1}{k} \approx \frac{1}{q} \int_{P}^{R(P)P} \frac{dx}{x}.$$

This sum can be approximated by the integral shown. The result is

$$E \approx \frac{1}{q} \log \frac{PR(P)}{P} = \frac{1}{q} \log R(P)$$

since the area under the curve $(1/q) \log R(P)$ is the sum plus an error that is no larger than $2/qP$, which is small if qP is large {see Ex. 1.10}.

By introducing the effort E, we have three variables, but only two equations

$$\begin{aligned} Y &= PR(P) - P \\ qE &= \log R(P). \end{aligned}$$

If it is possible to eliminate P from these equations, then a direct relationship between effort and yield will be found. The second equation gives

$$R(P) = \exp(qE).$$

Putting this in the first equation gives

$$P = Y/(\exp(qE) - 1)$$

and substituting this in the second equation gives

$$qE = \log R(Y/(\exp(qE) - 1))$$

or

$$\exp(qE) = R(Y/(\exp(qE) - 1)) \tag{1.5.1}$$

We must know the populations growth rate R in order to proceed. We consider three cases:

1. *Malthus's model.* In this case $R(P) = r$, so $Y = (r - 1)P$ and $E = (1/q) \log r$. There is no maximum sustained yield in this case. If $r > 1$, then the yield will be proportional to the standing stock P and it will require an effort $(1/q) \log r$ to produce it. If $r < 1$, then there is no sustained yield possible, reflecting the fact that the population is dying out.

2. *Verhulst's model.* In this case,

$$R(P) = r/(1 + P/K)$$

so

$$(rK \exp(-qE) - K) = Y/(\exp(qE) - 1)$$

or

$$Y = K(r \exp(-qE) - 1)(\exp(qE) - 1).$$

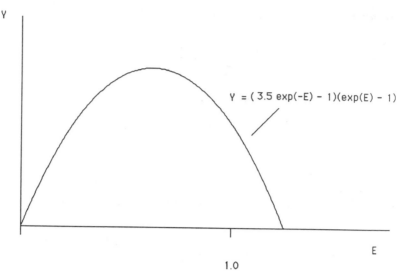

$$Y = (3.5 \exp(-E) - 1)(\exp(E) - 1)$$

1.0

FIGURE 1.10. Effort–yield curves for Verhulst's model.

Any effort that exceeds $(1/q) \log r$ would eliminate the population since then $Y < 0$. Moreover, the maximum sustained yield is obtained when $E^* = (1/2q) \log r$. These are plotted in Figure 1.10.

This calculation was carried out for fisheries by Beverton and Holt in 1957, and it led to the following policy for controlling a fishery. Effort is allowed to increase until a decrease in yield is observed. This means that E^* has been passed. Then effort is reduced until another decrease in yield is observed. This procedure is followed iteratively until the maximum sustained yield is reached.

3. *Ricker's model.* In this case, $R(P) = r \exp(-P/K)$, and

$$Y = (\log r - qE)(\exp(qE) - 1)K.$$

4. *Predator satiation model.* In this case, $R(P) = rP/(1 + P/K)$ and the yield-effort relation is

$$\exp(qE)(\exp(qE) - 1) = rY \exp(-Y/K(\exp(qE) - 1)).$$

As we have seen, the first two examples are straightforward. Ricker's model is included because we see that there is an optimal choice for effort to maintain a *sustained* maximum yield, but we know this model to have chaotic solutions when r is large. Because of this, it is certain that the sustained maximum will be unstable, and almost surely not be realizable.

The predator model illustrates another problem. Setting $z = Y/(\exp(qE) - 1)$, we get

$$\exp qE = rz \exp(-z/K).$$

The maximum of the right-hand side is rK/e, so for each E up to $E^{\#} = 1/q \log(r/e)$, there are two roots of the equation for z, say $z_1(E) < z_2(E)$.

They come together at $z = K$, so $z_1(E^{\#}) = z_2(E^{\#}) = K$. For larger values of E there are no sustained yields possible. The important point here is that if we allow E to increase until we see yields decline, the population can collapse before Y gets small, therefore, we run a significant risk of destroying the resource if we follow the strategy that worked for the Beverton–Holt fishery. The interval $E^{\#} - E^*$ gives the margin of safety in the management policy {see Ex. 1.10}.

1.6 Summary

Several approaches to modeling populations have been presented in this chapter. They will be repeated for various other population phenomena over the next three chapters. First, models based on difference equations were derived. We saw that in some cases, the models can be solved with an explicit formula for the solution that can be used as a basis for estimating parameters. In other cases, we found that the graphical cobwebbing method can be used to determine what happens to solutions. But, we studied some examples where neither method works. In those chaotic cases, we showed how various computer simulations can be used to describe how the solutions behave, even though they appear to be random. The histograms that we calculated in those examples will be seen again in the next three chapters where they appear as probability distributions. It is remarkable that nonrandom models like Ricker's can have solutions that must be described using words from probability theory.

We also saw several examples of differential equations approximating difference equations. This is based on considering the population problem using infinitesimal sampling intervals, and it is necessary for some studies where populations have overlapping generations. Some population problems, especially ones involving insects, are correctly modeled using difference equations. Still, the use of differential equations enables us to use calculus to find solution formulas that are not possible for difference equations. We will see this use of calculus arise repeatedly throughout the book.

The chapter began with a study of total population size and moved to a description of age structure in populations. Populations are stratified in many ways—by age, genetic types, mixing groups, etc., and accounting for stratification can be quite difficult. For one thing, much more data are required to make use of stratified models. For example, Malthus's model requires estimation of only one parameter, the growth rate b, but the renewal equation, which is the analogue of Malthus's model for age-structured populations, requires estimation of the age-specific birth and death rate functions $b(a)$ and $\lambda(a)$. However, in those cases, we found that the behavior was comparable—both populations grow exponentially. The exponential rate b in Malthus's case is the population's intrinsic growth, but the exponential rate r^* in the renewal equation depends on $b(a)$ and $\lambda(a)$ in subtle ways.

The last section presented some introductory work on harvesting, and it lays a basis for further reading and work in bioeconomics. The excellent book

[4] is recommended for further reading in this important area.

In the next several chapters, we will consider models in small populations and analogues in large populations, and we will see how the two situations are related

1.7 Annotated References

1. N. Keyfitz, and W. Flieger, *Population: Fact and methods of demography*, W. H. Freeman, San Francisco, 1971.

   An excellent source for demographic methods and data.

2. F. C. Hoppensteadt, *Mathematical methods of population biology*, Cambridge Univ. Press, New York, 1982.

   Presents many topics of this chapter in greater depth.

3. F.C. Hoppensteadt, *Mathematical theories of populations: Demographics, genetics and epidemics*, SIAM Publications, Philadelphia, 1975.

4. C. W. Clark, *Bioeconomics modeling and fishery management*, Wiley-Interscience, New York, 1985.

   An excellent introduction to the use of mathematics in resource management.

5. W. E. Ricker, *Stock and recruitment*, J. Fish. Res. Bd. Canada. **11** (1954), 559–623.

6. T.Y. Li and J.A. Yorke, *Period three implies chaos*, Amcr. Math. Monthly **82** (1975) 985–992.

   This paper introduced the word "chaos" to describe irregular behavior.

7. F. C. Hoppensteadt, and J.M. Hyman, *Periodic solutions to a discrete logistic equation*, SIAM J. Appl. Math. **32** (1977), 73–81.

Exercises

1.1. ESTIMATION OF HUMAN POPULATION GROWTH

a. Census data for Sweden collected at 20 year intervals are presented in Table 1.6.

Table 1.6. Swedish Population Data 1780–1860.

Year	Population (1000s)
1780	$2104 = P_{1780}$
1800	$2352 = P_{1800}$
1820	$2573 = P_{1820}$
1840	$3123 = P_{1840}$
1860	$3824 = P_{1860}$

Let P_n denote the population size in year n, and suppose that the model for this population is $P_{n+20} = r\, P_n$.

Use the least-squares method to show that $r = 1.6$.

Thus, the model becomes

$$P_{n+20} = 1.16 P_n.$$

This can be solved by starting with P_{1780} and marching forward: In general, K census intervals after 1780, we predict the population will be

$$P_{1780+20K} = (1.16)^K P_{1780}.$$

Compare the predicted values with those actually observed by completing Table 1.7.

Table 1.7. Swedish Population Data Projections 1780–1960.

Year	K	Observed	Predicted	% error
1780	0	2104	2104	0
1800	1	2352	2441	4
1820	2	2573	2831	10
1840	3	3123	3284	5
1860	4	3824	3810	0.5
1880	5	4572		
1900	6	5117		
1920	7	5876		
1940	8	6356		
1960	9	7480		

Here % error $= 100$(observed - predicted)/predicted.

b. Plot the observed Swedish population data in Table 1.7 in pairs (P_n, P_{n+20}). Use the least-squares method to fit a straight line to these data. Compare this answer with the result of 1.1.a.

1.2. GENERALIZATION OF FIBONACCI'S EQUATION

Consider the recursion

$$R_{n+1} = a\,R_n + b\,R_{n-1}$$

with $R_0 = 1$ and $R_1 = 1$. For what values of a and b does $R_n \to 0$? What happens in the other cases?

1.3. RICKER'S MODEL

a. Reproduce the results in Tables 1.2, 1.3, 1.4, and 1.5.

b. Carry out Tables 1.4 and 1.5 using the same program but for 300 intervals and 30,000 iterations. Plot the histogram for $r = 10.0$ and $r = 20.0$.

c. Repeat the calculation in 1.3.b for several values of r to investigate various parts of Figure 1.5.

1.4. OTHER CHAOTIC MAPPINGS

a. Consider the reproduction function

$$P_{n+1} = rP_n/(1 + P_n^M).$$

Describe the solutions of this iteration for every fixed value of the constant integer M.

b. Consider the reproduction function

$$P_{n+1} = r\,P_n(1 - P_n/K)$$

with $P_o = 0.5$ and $0 \le P_n \le K$. Describe the behavior of its solutions for various values of $r, 0 \le r \le 4$, by calculating and plotting iteration histograms.

c. Note that when $r = 4$, a solution can be found. [Hint: Let $P_n = \sin^2 \theta_n$. Then $\sin^2 \theta_{n+1} = 4\sin^2 \theta_n \cos^2 \theta_n = \sin^2 2\,\theta_n$. Therefore, $\theta_n = 2^n \theta_o$ (modulo 2π) {see Ex. 1.6}.]

1.5. ENTROPY

a. Show that the entropy function $H(f_1, f_2, ..., f_N)$ has the properties listed in Section 1.3.3.

b. Find all distributions (p_1, p_2, p_3) $(N = 3)$ for which $H = 1.0$, and for which $H = \log 2 / \log 3$, and plot them on triangular coordinates. That is, draw an equilateral triangle having altitude 1. Label the vertices 1, 2, and 3. A point (p_1, p_2, p_3) with $p_i \geq 0$ and $p_1 + p_2 + p_3 = 1$ can be located at a unique point of this graph by moving p_1 units away from the side opposite vertex 1, p_2 units away from the side opposite the vertex 2, and p_3 units away from the side opposite the vertex 3. These lines intersect at one point since the vertical distances add up to the altitude of the triangle. We will use these triangular coordinates in other applications in Section 2.4.

1.6. A STRANGE ATTRACTOR

Consider the xy-plane written in polar coordinates:

$$r = \sqrt{(x^2 + y^2)}, \theta = \tan^{-1} y/x, \quad \text{so} \quad 0 \leq r < \infty \quad \text{and} \quad 0 \leq \theta < 2\pi.$$

The inverse relation is $x = r \cos \theta$ and $y = r \sin \theta$.

a. Consider the following mapping of the plane into itself,

$$r_{n+1} = r_n e^{1-r_n}, \quad \theta_{n+1} = 2\,\theta_n \quad (\text{modulo} \quad 2\pi).$$

Show that all iterates approach the unit circle $r = 1$. (That is, show that $r_n \to 1$ as $n \to \infty$.) The unit circle is invariant under this mapping in the sense that if the iteration starts on it, it stays on it. On the unit circle, we need only study the mapping $\theta_{n+1} = 2\theta_n$ modulo 2π of the circle into itself. Show that there is a solution of period 2^N for any integer N. (Hint: $\theta_n = 2^n \theta_0$ modulo 2π. Find $\theta_0 \neq 0$ so $\theta_N = 2^N \theta_0 = \theta_0$ modulo 2π.)

b. Draw the graph $\theta_{n+1} = 2\,\theta_n$ modulo 2π by plotting θ_{n+1} versus θ_n. Try to find a periodic orbit by cobwebbing. Use the histogram method to study this mapping of the circle onto itself.

c. Show that there are initial points θ_o that lead to iterations that never repeat themselves.

These calculations show that the unit circle is an attractor, and that behavior of iterates on the attractor is quite irregular, having periodic and aperiodic iterations hopelessly intertwined. Such a set is referred to as being a strange attractor.

1.7. THE LOGISTIC EQUATION

a. Show that if $r = 1 + bh$ and h is small, then the difference equation

$$P_{n+1} = r\, P_n/(1 + (P_n/K))$$

and the differential equation

$$\frac{dp}{dt} = b\, p\, \left(1 - \frac{p}{K}\right)$$

are close by estimating $P_n - p(nh)$.

b. Show that a differential equation

$$\frac{dp}{dt} = F(p)$$

where F is a continuously differentiable function must have all solutions monotone (that is, either constant, strictly increasing or strictly decreasing). Conclude that it cannot have chaotic, or even periodic, solutions.

1.8. CHEMOSTAT POPULATION DYNAMICS

A chemostat is a continuous culture device used for growing and studying bacteria. Nutrient is added at a constant rate, say $S_0 \lambda$ (Mass/Volume)(Volume/Time), to the growth chamber where living cells are stirred in the enriched media. The growth chamber is continually adjusted to keep a constant volume by removing fluid at the flow rate λ. Let $S(t)$ denote the concentration of nutrient in the growth chamber at time t, and let $B(t)$ denote the concentration of bacteria.

The mathematical model for the chemostat uses the Jacob-Monod model in (1.3.4) and accounts for the addition of nutrient and the washing out of cells:

$$\frac{dS}{dt} = \lambda(S_0 - S(t)) - \frac{VSB}{K+S}\frac{1}{Y}$$

$$\frac{dB}{dt} = \frac{VSB}{K+S} - \lambda B$$

where λ is the flow rate, V is the maximum uptake rate, K is the saturation constant of nutrient uptake and Y is the yield of cells per unit nutrient taken up.

Determine the optimal flow rate for keeping the cells in their exponential growth phase. Show that if λ is too large, then the population washes out.

1.9. PERIODICAL CICADAS

Consider a population of cicadas that have a life-span of L years. Let X_n denote the number of newborns that become established underground in year n. Let α denote the probability of survival underground per year, and let P denote a predator satiation threshold. Then the number of cicadas that emerge L years later is $X_n \alpha^L$. The remainder of these after predator satiation can be denoted by

$E_n = (X_{n+L} \alpha^L - P)_+ =$ number of adults emerging in year $n + L$. Here the notation $(h)_+$ equals h if $h \geq 0$ and is zero otherwise. If each of these survivors bears b viable offspring, then $H_n = bE_n$ gives the number of newborns that could become established underground in year $n + L$.

However, the environmental carrying capacity might limit this. If K is the carrying capacity for developing cicadas, the residual carrying capacity is

$$K_n = (K - \sum_{j=1}^{L-1} X_{n-j}\alpha^j)_+.$$

Therefore, the number of offspring becoming established underground in year $n + L$ is

$$X_{n+L} = \min\{H_n, K_n\}.$$

a. Show that the population becomes extinct unless $b\,\alpha^L > 1$.

b. Suppose that L is a composite integer ($L = pq$ where p and q are integers). Determine conditions on b, α, P, K, and L that ensure that there can be a p-periodic emergence pattern. That is, show that under certain conditions on the data there is a solution of the form $X_{N_p} = X$ for $N = 1, 2, \ldots$, but $X_j = 0$ if j is not a multiple of p.

1.10. EFFORT–YIELD CURVES FOR HARVESTING

Plot the yield–effort curves for the two cases of Ricker's model and the predator satiation model as derived in Section 1.5. Discuss the possible results of the maximum sustained yield management policy in these two cases.

1.11*. PROJECT ON POPULATION SIMULATION

Write and execute a computer program for solving the renewal equation (1.2.2), and so calculate the sequence $\{B_n\}$ using the data $\lambda_n = (0.95)^n$, $b_n = 0$ if $n \leq 15$, and $b_n = 1.1$ for $16 \leq n \leq 30$, and beyond that $b_n = 1.1(0.8)^n$. Let $h_n = 0$ for all n, but $B_0 = 1.0$.

a. Calculate the numbers $B_1, \ldots, B_{150}$.

b. Plot successive age histograms (see Figure 1.1) for the total female population size at every fifth sampling interval by calculating the number of individuals of each age group.

c. Calculate the value of r^* as described in the Renewal Theorem.

d. Plot the successive age histograms for $r^{*-n}B_n$. These converge to what is known as the *stable age distribution* of the population.

1.12*. A Project on Leslie's Matrix

A matrix formulation of Fibonacci's model is possible. Let $\mathbf{v}_n = (R_n, R_{n-1})$, for $n = 1, 2, \ldots$, and let

$$\mathbf{E} = \begin{pmatrix} 1 & 1 \\ 1 & 0 \end{pmatrix}.$$

a. Show that Fibonacci's model is equivalent to the iteration

$$\mathbf{v}_{n+1} = \mathbf{v}_n\mathbf{E}.$$

b. Find the eigenvalues of $\mathbf{E}$. Use the solution for R_n in section 1.2.1 to find $\mathbf{v}_n$. Rewrite your answer in terms of the eigenvalues of $\mathbf{E}$. This method illustrates the spectral method for solving matrix iterations, which will be carried out in greater detail in Exercise 2.8.

1.13*. Laplace's Method for Solving the Renewal Equation

Consider Equation (1.2.4), the renewal equation, when there are overlapping generations.

$$B(t) = h(t) + \int_0^t b(a)\lambda(a)B(t-a)da.$$

Look for solutions of the homogeneous renewal equation (i.e., $h = 0$) in the form

$$B(t) = e^{rt}.$$

The result on substituting this into the equation is

$$1 = \int_0^\infty b(a)\lambda(a)e^{-ra}da.$$

This equation is difficult to solve for r. However, let $b(a)\lambda(a) = B$ for $15 < a < 30$ and otherwise be zero. Then the equation becomes

$$\frac{r}{B} = e^{-15r} - e^{-30r}.$$

a. Find the largest value of r that satisfies this equation. (Hint: Find where the right hand side has a maximum value and determine for what values of b, the straight line r/B can cross the curve on the right.)

b. The solution of this equation has the form $B(t) \propto e^{r^*t} +$ smaller terms so show that $e^{-r^*t}B(t) \to A$ as $t \to \infty$. This is the stable birth rate.

c. Determine the population's age distribution when $B(t) = A\,e^{r^*t}$.

2

Inheritance

Genetics is the study of heredity and variation among organisms. The initial breakthroughs in genetics came with observations made by Darwin and Mendel in the 19th century, and mathematics came to play an important role in bringing us to our present-day understanding of genetics. Work in the first half of the 20th century by J.B.S. Haldane, S. Wright, R.A. Fisher, and others put this important area of biology on a firm mathematical base that helped in the design and interpretation of experiments. Many think that genetics still represents the outstanding application of mathematics in the life sciences.

It is known that in all living organisms, reproduction involves the passing from one generation to the next a genetic code that determines all physical aspects of the offspring. This code is carried on chromosomes. *Chromosomes* are large molecules in living cells that carry the information for all of its chemical needs. Some human cells (sperm and eggs) have single chromosomes, but most other cells in the body have chromosomes occurring in matched pairs. Plants can have chromosomes appearing in matched sets of three or four or more. When a single chromosome occurs, the cell is called a *haploid cell.* It is a *diploid* cell if the chromosomes occur in matched pairs, and a *polyploid* cell otherwise. Human diploid cells have 23 chromosome pairs that are arranged like strands stuck together near their centers. Bacteria are haploid cells having a single chromosome that is arranged in a closed loop.

Genes are segments of a chromosome that code for some specific (identifiable) cell function, such as the production of a protein molecule. The location of a gene is called its *locus.* The gene may appear in several slightly variant forms within a population that are detectable by experiments. These variants are called *alleles.* While the genetic code has been broken showing how the chemical structure of chromosomes correlates with amino acids, the basic building blocks of proteins, the complicated spatial configuration of chromosomes, has blocked detection of most genes [see 1].

Genetics encompasses all the studies of genes in all plants and animals. It has been an active and interesting area of work over the past century. Genetic studies have given us tools to understand and reduce diseases, they have resulted in important social, political, and legal decisions and policies, they have made possible the development of entirely novel organisms that are important in agriculture, biotechnology, and medicine, and they stimulated the growth of new sciences. For example, the study of genetics contributed to the foundations of probability theory and mathematical statistics as derived by Fisher, Haldane, and Wright [see 2]. The genome project being undertaken by the United States government underscores the importance of this area to our lives. The project is attempting to map all chromosomes carried by humans.

Three important problems are presented in this chapter, and each is solved using different mathematical tools. The first problem is to describe natural selection for a simple genetic trait. We consider a gene locus having two alleles, and we use Mendel's laws to construct a model for how the distribution of genes in a large population can change.

Second, we consider antibiotic resistance in bacteria, and we study how pure resistant strains are created through random genetic drift. This introduces the use of random models, namely Markov chains, to understand how uncertain events can have long-range influence. As a rough guide, when a population involves fewer than 30 individuals, random events can have great effect, but in larger populations random fluctuations balance each other [3]. A similar calculation describes how a genetic mutation in a small human population could take over and become established.

It is quite an impressive intellectual step to account for small random fluctuations and still derive a sensible theory to guide experiments and theory. The key concept is that of probability: We can characterize tossing a fair coin by the number $\frac{1}{2}$. There are two possible outcomes (heads or tails) and in a great many throws, we will see approximately one half of them being heads. We say the probability of heads is $1/2$. Of course, the probability of tails is $1 - \frac{1}{2} = \frac{1}{2}$. However, this number does not capture many important aspects of these experiments, such as what can be said about the results of a fixed number of experiments, but it is an important start.

It is frequently observed that a simple relation exists between the numbers of various genotypes in a population. These are referred to as Hardy–Weinberg proportions. We study the stability of genetic systems, including the Hardy–Weinberg proportions, in Section 2.4.

2.1   Mendel's Laws

Let us consider a diploid population and denote two possible alleles at a certain locus by **a** and **b**. Individuals can be genetically typed by their genes at this locus: they are either **aa**, **ab** or **bb** (note that **ab** and **ba** are indistinguishable here). These are called *genotypes*. In the case of the blood disease sickle cell anemia, the **b** gene might code for the anemic trait, and those of type **bb** will have the disease. Those of types **aa** and **ab** do not have the disease, although the offspring of those of type **ab** are at risk of inheriting two **b** genes from an **ab** × **ab** mating, and so inherit the disease.

The whole population carries a pool of genes at the locus under consideration, and by studying the gene pool we can make certain predictions about the fate of, say, the **b** gene in the population. This is done in the following way. First, to avoid the (minor) complications of overlapping generations, we consider a synchronized population, and we attempt to describe the changes

TABLE 2.1. Mendel's laws.

Parents	Progeny		
	aa	**ab**	**bb**
aa × **aa**	1		
aa × **ab**	1/2	1/2	
aa × **bb**		1	
ab × **ab**	1/4	1/2	1/4
ab × **bb**		1/2	1/2
bb × **bb**			1

that will occur in the gene pool with each reproduction.

The gene pool is described from one generation to the next by the sequence $\{g_n\}$ where g_n denotes the proportion of the gene pool that is of type **a** immediately before the nth reproduction. The reproduction process creates a new population whose genes are selected from the parent's gene pool at random according to Mendel's laws. These laws summarize observations of the reproduction of plant genes made by Gregor Mendel in 1850. The laws are summarized in Table 2.1 where, for example, one parent of type **aa** mated with a parent of type **bb** will produce offspring of type **ab**, but the offspring of an **ab** mated with an **ab** will be $\frac{1}{4}$ **aa**, $\frac{1}{4}$ **bb** and $\frac{1}{2}$ **ab** offspring on the average.

Creation of a new generation by its parents can be viewed as a random process. A population of N individuals carries $2N$ genes in its pool, and the distribution of their reproductive haploid cells at reproduction time gives the probabilities of various ones being used in reproduction. For example, the proportion of the offspring who are of type **aa** will be

$$g_n^2 + g_n(1 - g_n) \tag{2.1.1}$$

since the probability of two **a** genes being selected for reproduction will be $g_n \times g_n$, and the probability of one **a** and one **b** gene being selected will be $2g_n(1 - g_n)$, half of which will be **a** genes.

The fitnesses of various offspring are like the numbers in the renewal equation in Chapter 1. They describe probability of survival to the next reproduction time and fertility. These will be denoted by the numbers R for **aa**, S for **ab**, and T for **bb** types of offspring. Therefore, the total gene pool at the next reproduction time will be proportional to

$$w_n = R\,g_n^2 + 2\,S\,g_n(1 - g_n) + T(1 - g_n)^2$$

and those of type **a** will be proportional to

$$R\,g_n^2 + S\,g_n(1 - g_n)$$

as in Equation (2.1.1). Therefore, the gene pool proportion of type **a** at the next reproduction is determined by the formula

$$g_{n+1} = \frac{R\, g_n^2 + S g_n(1 - g_n)}{w_n}. \tag{2.1.2}$$

The changes in the gene pool through the generations can be determined by iterating this relation as described in several examples in Chapter 1. Four typical cases are shown in Figure 2.1

The four cases described in Figure 2.1 require a little bit of mathematical analysis to uncover, but they have simple interpretations. In case a, $R > S > T$, and the **a** gene is favored. It will eventually dominate the gene pool since $g_n \to 1$. This is the situation for sickle cell disease in the United States where **b** is the anemic gene. In case b, $R < S < T$, and **b** wins. The remaining two cases are of particular interest. Heterosis occurs if the mixed type **ab** has a higher probability of surviving and reproducing than the two pure types **aa** and **bb**. For example, in sickle cell disease in tropical climates the **aa** types are not anemic, but they are at higher risk of contracting malaria than the other two types. The **bb** type has the sickle cell trait and so is at risk from it. Figure 2.1C therefore shows that the gene **b**, which is the deleterious one in an environment having no malaria, is maintained by the disease in other climates. The final case Figure 2.1D is difficult to document in the field, but it is believed to be an important mechanism in the process of speciation and evolutionary divergence of species.

The model (2.1.2) was derived by Fisher, Wright, and Haldane in the 1930s, and it has been widely used to study genetic traits. The model is based on the gene pool that is available at reproduction time. The gene pool is not observable in most populations, but rather the genotypes of the organisms often can be determined directly. The population comprises the genotypes **aa**, **ab** and **bb**, and these can frequently be identified, for example, using electrophoretic methods of biochemistry.

If there is no selective difference between the genotypes, then $R = S = T$, and we have that

$$g_{n+1} = \frac{g_n^2 + g_n(1 - g_n)}{g_n^2 + 2g_n(1 - g_n) + (1 - g_n)^2} = g_n. \tag{2.1.3}$$

Therefore, the genotype proportions in the nth generation satisfy

$$\mathbf{aa : ab : bb} = g_n^2 : 2g_n(1 - g_n) : (1 - g_n)^2 = g_o^2 : 2g_o(1 - g_o) : (1 - g_o)^2$$

and the population is said to be in *Hardy–Weinberg* proportions. This observation was purportedly made by the mathematician G.H. Hardy during a tennis game and independently by the German physician W. Weinberg {see Ex. 2.1}. We will study these proportions when there is selection in Section 2.4.

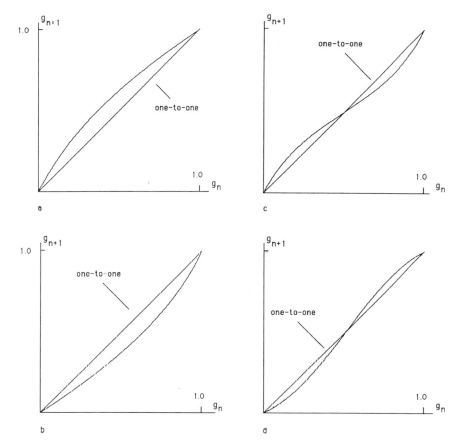

FIGURE 2.1. **A**, **a** dominates, $R > S > T$. **b**, **B** dominates $R < S < T$. **c**, *Heterosis*, $S > R, S > T$. **d**, *Disruptive selection*, $S < R, S < T$.

2.2   Bacterial Genetics: Plasmids

The biological problems described in this section are ones from genetic engineering, and they are concerned with a mechanism used to introduce new genes into a bacterium to cause it to perform a specific function, such as the production of a particular enzyme. In this section we derive a model that accounts for random sampling of the gene pool at each reproduction. Obviously, since the reproduction involves randomness at each step, we cannot predict exactly how the population will evolve. Instead, we derive what the statistical distribution of many similar populations will be. The model that results is called a Markov chain. Several examples of Markov chains will be studied here and in Chapters 3 and 4.

The genetic system that we study here is simpler than the one in the preceding section—we consider bacteria that are haploid organisms. Bacteria are single-celled organisms that are enclosed within a cell wall; the interior is made up of cytoplasmic material and it contains the various mechanisms needed for cell life and reproduction. In particular, the chromosome is a circular loop of *DNA* (deoxyribonucleic acid) that carries a code for all cell functions, as opposed to pairs of linear chromosomes described in the preceding section for diploids. As described earlier, a gene is a segment of the chromosome that codes for production, such as of an enzyme or another protein.

Many types of bacteria have additional genetic material called extrachromosomal DNA elements or *plasmids*. Plasmids are small circular pieces of DNA that also carry genes. However, plasmids can pass from cell to cell, and some genes can "jump" from plasmids to chromosomes, and in this way become permanently incorporated in the cell's code.

The cell cycle begins with a newborn daughter. All of the cell's components, including the chromosome and plasmids (if any are present), are copied during the replication phase. The replication is followed by splitting or division of the cell into two daughters, each receiving one replicate of the chromosome.

In this section, we study how drug resistance is passed vertically through generations of bacteria by the mechanism of random genetic drift.

We consider a plasmid P that appears in two forms, say P' and P''. These two forms differ perhaps at just a few points on their DNA, but otherwise they are entirely similar. For example, P' could carry a gene that codes for *resistance* of the cell to the antibiotic ampicillin and P'' could code for resistance to tetracycline.

The purpose here is to predict the fate of the two plasmid types P' and P'' in the cell line after many generations.

The plasmid P is assumed to appear with N copies in all newborn cells and to replicate according to a cycle depicted by the graph

$$
\begin{array}{ccccc}
 & \text{replication} & & \text{partitioning} & \\
N & \longrightarrow & 2N & \longrightarrow & N
\end{array}
$$

We suppose for simplicity that the division cycle of all cells is synchronized throughout the population, and that the copy number N is constant for all cells.

At each cell division there is a random distribution of plasmids among the two daughters. As a result of this, there can be a great number of possible evolutions of a cell colony. This phenomenon is referred to as *random genetic drift* since genetic types change, but as a result of random sampling rather than natural selection or other forces.

A model of plasmid dynamics is formulated in the following way: Let $p_i =$ proportion of newborn cells having iP'−plasmids and $N-i$ P''−plasmids. After replication, there will be $2N$ plasmids, $2i$ of them will be of type P' and $2N-2i$ of type P''.

There are a number of ways that these $2N$ plasmids can be distributed among the two daughters, and the theory of probability tells how to count the possibilities. We suppose that each daughter receives N copies. Of these, j copies of P' can be selected for one daughter in

$$\binom{2i}{j}$$

different ways. The notation

$$\binom{m}{n}$$

is the usual binomial coefficient, where

$$\binom{m}{n} = \frac{m!}{n!(m-n)!}$$

The total number of partitions is

$$\binom{2N}{N}$$

and the number of ways one daughter can have jP' and $N-jP''$ plasmids is

$$\binom{2i}{j}\binom{2N-2i}{N-j}$$

if the mother originally had iP' and $N-iP''$ plasmids. Therefore, the formula

$$P_{i,j} = \frac{\binom{2i}{j}\binom{2N-2i}{N-j}}{\binom{2N}{N}}$$

gives the probability of one daughter having jP' and $N-jP''$ plasmids. That is, if very many observations were made of such reproductions, then this is the proportion that would have one daughter having jP' and the other having $N-jP''$ plasmids.

TABLE 2.2. Sample Calculation for $N = 4, p_2^{(o)} = 1$

Time	$\mathbf{p}^n$				
$n = 0$	0.0	0.0	1.0	0.0	0.0
$n = 1$	0.01	0.23	0.51	0.23	0.01
$n = 2$	0.06	0.25	0.37	0.25	0.06
$n = 40$	0.5	0.0	0.0	0.0	0.5

Based on these calculations, we can determine the evolution of the plasmid distributions in an interesting way. The population in a given generation can be described by the vector $\mathbf{p} = (p_o, p_1, ..., p_N)$, which tells the proportions of the various cell types appearing in the population. Let us denote these numbers in the next generation by $q_o, q_1, ..., q_N$, respectively. Then

$$q_j = p_o P_{o,j} + p_1 P_{1,j} + ... + p_N P_{N,j} \quad \text{for} \quad j = 0, ..., N,$$

This states that the proportion of cells having jP' plasmids next generation is the sum of the proportion having zero now times the probability of leaving j plasmids starting from none, plus the proportion of cells having one now times the probability of leaving j starting from one, etc. Using matrix notation, we write this more concisely as

$$\mathbf{q} = \mathbf{p}\,\mathbf{P}$$

where we set $\mathbf{q} = (q_o, ..., q_N)$. This recursion scheme is not difficult to analyze and use. If $\mathbf{p} = \mathbf{p}^{(n)}$ is the distribution in the nth generation, then $\mathbf{q} = \mathbf{p}^{(n+1)}$ and so using the back substitution method we have that

$$\mathbf{p}^{(n)} = \mathbf{p}^{(o)}\mathbf{P}^n. \tag{2.2.1}$$

This recursion, called a *Markov Chain*, is one of the basic tools in studies of random processes. It is named in honor of the 19th century Russian mathematician A. A. Markov who derived this method while studying probabilities in playing-card games. The ideas were taken up in this century by Fisher and others who applied them to many genetics problems. In fact, Fisher's work laid the foundation of the modern mathematical theory of genetics in plants and animals.

The numbers in Table 2.2 show the evolution of the population proportions for a population that starts out having two of four plasmids of type P'.

Note that the model (2.2.1) has no randomness in it. Once $\mathbf{p}^{(o)}$ is known, all the vectors $\mathbf{p}^{(n)}$ are uniquely determined by the formula. The components of $\mathbf{p}^{(n)}$ give the proportions of the population having various plasmid combinations at the nth sampling. That is, $p_{j,n}$, which is the jth component of $\mathbf{p}^{(n)}$, gives the probability that at the nth sampling a cell having j P' plasmids would be selected from the population as a sample.

These data demonstrate a very important phenomenon. After many generations, the population is divided (almost) equally between those having all P' plasmids and those having all P'' plasmids, and neither is resistant to both antibiotics, as was the original population! It was thought for many years that there was an interaction between plasmids of different type that drove them apart so that only one could be present in a cell at one time without there being the external force of selection. This phenomenon was called *plasmid instability*. However, we see from the calculation just done that it can be simple random sampling at each division time that is responsible for plasmid instability. In rough terms, if a cell is purely one type or the other, all of its daughters will be also, and we say that the cell is in an *absorbing state* with respect to this plasmid type. Any other distribution of the two plasmids has a chance to change at each division, and so they eventually will. The absorbing states always win!

Changes in the genetic profile of a population due simply to random sampling of genes at reproduction time is referred to as *random genetic drift*, and it is believed to play an important role in the evolution of species. The mathematical analysis of Markov chain models provides an explanation for these facts, which are actually observed to occur in bacterial experiments {see Ex. 2.2 and 2.8}.

The issue of stability of plasmids in cell lines is quite an important one since in biotechnology cells are instructed to produce certain materials by insertion of a plasmid carrying the instructions as genetic code. It is important that the plasmid stay in the cell line to ensure that production continues. Problems of this kind are just now being solved [4].

2.3 Genetics in Small Populations of Humans

As we have seen, creation of one generation by its parents can be viewed as a random process. For a one-locus, two-allele genetic trait, a population of N humans carries $2N$ genes, and the distribution of their gametes at reproduction time gives the probabilities of various ones being used in reproduction. For example, the offspring of a population consisting of one male and one female that produce two offspring are summarized in Table 2.3.

Table 2.3 shows that with probability $1/8(= \frac{1}{16} + \frac{1}{16})$, one of the alleles is entirely lost from the population! Moreover, with probability $1/4$ there are no heterozygotes in the population. Therefore, random genetic drift can cause quite important changes in the population's genetic structure.

The gene pool of the next generation is formed by sampling the adult gamete pool. In the first section of this chapter, we considered a large population and took the expected numbers to make the model. In a small population, we must account for all possible events, like we did for bacteria and in Table 2.3.

Let the alleles be denoted by **a** and **b**, and let α_n denote the number of **a** genes in the nth generation. Then $p_n = \alpha_n/2N$ gives the frequency of **a** genes in the gene pool. The population is assumed to mate at random and be

TABLE 2.3. Two Offspring of Two **ab**'s

Type of Offspring		
One Offspring	The Other One	Probability
aa	**aa**	1/16
ab	**aa**	$1/8 + 1/8 = 1/4$
ab	**ab**	1/4
bb	**ab**	1/4
bb	**bb**	1/16
aa	**bb**	1/8

synchronized with nonoverlapping generations. Furthermore, the population size is assumed to remain constant through the generations.

The sequence of random variables $\{\alpha_n\}$ describes the offspring gene pool immediately after reproduction in successive generations. If α_n is known, then α_{n+1} has a *binomial distribution* (sampling with replacement) with parameter $p_n = \alpha_n/2N$ and index $2N$. In particular, at the end of the nth reproduction period the gene pool consists of α_n **a** genes and $2N - \alpha_n$ **b** genes. The probability that $\alpha_{n+1} = j$ in the next generation given that $\alpha_n = i$ is

$$
P_{i,j} = Pr[\alpha_{n+1} = j \mid \alpha_n = i] = \binom{2N}{j} \left(\frac{i}{2N}\right)^j \left(1 - \frac{i}{2N}\right)^{2N-j} .
$$

The matrix $\mathbf{P} = (P_{ij})$ defines a Markov chain for simple human genetic traits. This is called the *Fisher–Wright* chain. We can use it as we did the plasmid chain to determine the distribution of the population after many generations. Rather than pursuing this here, we consider a similar problem in epidemics in Chapter 3 {see Ex. 2.3}.

2.4   The Hardy–Weinberg Equilibrium

Difference equations and Markov chains have some limitations. For example, although it is reasonably easy to derive models using them, it is often difficult to derive formulas that describe the eventual evolution of their solutions. Calculus provides important methods for solving such problems. Therefore, it is of some interest to derive genetics models in the form of differential equations.

Consider a one-locus, two allele genetic trait in a large population as in Section 2.1. The alleles are denoted by **a** and **b**, and the possible genotypes are **aa**, **ab**, and **bb**. Instead of accounting for discrete generations, we will consider the case of overlapping generations where the sampling interval is very short. We suppose that the selective differences are small over a short time interval of length h:

$$R = 1 + h\,\rho, S = 1 + h\,\sigma, T = 1 + h\,\tau$$

where ρ, σ, and τ are some numbers and h is the sampling interval. Using this in formula (2.1.1) gives

$$g_{n+1} = \frac{g_n + h(\rho g_n + \sigma\, g_n(1 - g_n))}{1 + hW_n}$$

where $W_n = \rho\, g_n^2 + 2\,\sigma\, g_n(1 - g_n) + \tau(1 - g_n)^2$. Expanding this expression in powers of h gives

$$g_{n+1} = g_n + h(\rho g_n + \sigma g_n(1 - g_n) - g_n W_n) + O(h^2)$$

The notation $O(h^2)$ indicates terms that are of size h^2. We try to find a smooth function $p(t)$ such that $g_n = p(nh)$ when h is small. Rearranging terms and setting $t = nh$ in this formula gives

$$\frac{p(t + h) - p(t)}{h} = \rho p^2 + \sigma p(1 - p) - p(\rho p^2 + 2\sigma p(1 - p) + \tau(1 - p)^2) + O(h)$$

This is approximated by the differential equation

$$\frac{dp}{dt} = \rho p^2 + \sigma p(1 - p) - p(\rho p^2 + 2\sigma p(1 - p) + \tau(1 - p)^2)$$

or

$$\frac{dp}{dt} = p(1 - p)((\rho - 2\sigma + \tau)p + \sigma - \tau) \tag{2.4.1}$$

We will justify this approximation later. However, note that if the values in Figure 2.1 are used, we get similar results. That is, $\rho > \sigma > \tau$ implies that $p \to 1$, etc. {see Ex 2.4}.

If the population were in Hardy–Weinberg proportions, we would have **aa** : **ab** : **bb** $= p^2 : 2p(1 - p) : (1 - p)^2$. But, what are the proportions when there is selection? Do Hardy–Weinberg proportions prevail? To answer these questions, we derive a model for the *genotype* frequencies.

Let $x(t), 2y(t)$, and $z(t)$ be the numbers of **aa**, **ab**, and **bb** individuals in the population at time t, respectively, and let their birth rates be b_1, b_2, and b_3 and their death rates be d_1, d_2, and d_3, respectively. Finally, the total population will be denoted by $P(t)$ where

$$P(t) = x(t) + 2y(t) + z(t).$$

As before, $p(t)$ will denote the proportion of the gene pool that is of type **a**. The factor of 2 in the y term of P is used as in Section 2.1 for convenience in counting heterozygotes.

We will derive equations for x, y, z, and p. The gene pool at time t has size

$$2(x + 2y + z) = 2P$$

since each individual carries two genes at the locus, and in the gene pool are $2x + 2y$ **a** genes and $2y + 2z$ **b** genes. The proportion of the gene pool that is of type **a** is

$$p = (x + y)/P$$

and the proportion that is of type **b** is

$$q = (y + z)/P.$$

(Note that $p + q = 1$.) $b_1 \, dt$ is the number of offspring to each of the **aa**'s in a short time interval of length dt. Similarly, the births to **ab** and **bb** parents are $2y \, b_2 \, dt$ and $z \, b_3 \, dt$, respectively. The number of deaths of **aa**, **ab**, and **bb** individuals are $x \, d_1 \, dt, 2y \, d_2 \, dt$, and $z \, d_3 \, dt$, respectively. Then

$$\frac{dx}{dt} \quad = \quad (\# \text{ births to } \mathbf{aa})(\text{proportion fertilized by } \mathbf{a})$$

$$+ \quad \frac{1}{2} \, (\# \text{ births to } \mathbf{ab})(\text{proportion fertilized by } \mathbf{a}) \text{ - deaths}$$

so

$$dx = (b_1 \, x \frac{x + y}{x + 2y + z} + \frac{b_2 2y}{2} \frac{x + y}{x + 2y + z} - d_1 \, x) dt$$

etc.

Rearranging terms shows that

$$\frac{dx}{dt} \quad = \quad (b_1 x + b_2 y)p - d_1 x$$

$$2 \frac{dy}{dt} \quad = \quad (b_1 x + b_2 y)q + (b_3 \, z + b_2 y)p - d_2 \, 2y$$

$$\frac{dz}{dt} \quad = \quad (b_3 \, z + b_2 y)q - d_3 \, z.$$

These appear to be quite complicated equations, but several interesting things can be said about them without much effort.

The next step in our derivation is to consider the proportions of the total population that are **aa**, **ab** and **bb** genotypes. We denote them by D, $2H$, and R, respectively. This notation is useful if one thinks of dominant (**aa**), heterozygous (**ab**), and recessive (**bb**), although these designations are not correct under all selection schemes. In any case, we set

$$D = x/P, \; 2H = 2y/P, \; R = z/P$$

and it follows that {Ex. 2.6}

$$\frac{dD}{dt} = \frac{dx/dt}{P} - \frac{x}{P} \frac{dP/dt}{P} = (b_1 D + b_2 H)p - d_1 D - \overline{m} \, D$$

$$2 \frac{dH}{dt} = (b_1 D + b_2 H)q + (b_3 R + b_2 H)p - 2d_2 H - \overline{m} \, 2H \qquad (2.4.2)$$

$$\frac{dR}{dt} = (b_3 R + b_2 H)q - d_3 R - \overline{m}\, R$$

where $p = D + H$ and $q = R + H$ and

$$\overline{m} = \frac{dP/dt}{P} = (b_1 - d_1)D + 2(b_2 - d_2)H + (b_3 - d_3)R.$$

This term is referred to as the mean fitness of the population. Since $p = D + H$, an equation for p can be found by adding the first equation in (2.4.2) to half the second one. The result is

$$\frac{dp}{dt} = (m_1 - \overline{m})p$$

where

$$m_1 = b_1 D \frac{p+1}{2p} + b_2 H \frac{2p+1}{2p} + \frac{b_3 R}{2} - \frac{d_1 D}{P} - \frac{d_2 H}{P}.$$

m_1 is referred to as being the marginal fitness of allele **a**.

We first show that this population is in Hardy–Weinberg proportions if and only if

$$H^2 = DR. \tag{2.4.3}$$

To see this, first observe that if the Hardy–Weinberg proportions hold, then there is a common factor α such that $D = \alpha p^2$, $2H = \alpha 2pq$, and $R = \alpha q^2$. Then $DR = (\alpha pq)^2 = H^2$. On the other hand, if $H^2 = DR$, then since $p = D + H$ and $q = H + R$,

$$p^2 = D^2 + 2\,DH + H^2 = D^2 + 2DH + DR = D(D + 2H + R) = D$$

and similarly for $2pq$ and q^2. Formula (2.4.3) is a useful test for Hardy–Weinberg proportions {Ex. 2.7}.

No selection: Let us first check that Equation (2.4.2) is consistent with our earlier work when there is no selection: We suppose that there are numbers b and d such that

$$b_1 = b_2 = b_3 = b \quad \text{and} \quad d_1 = d_2 = d_3 = d.$$

Then,

$$\overline{m} = b - d$$

and

$$\frac{dD}{dt} = b(p^2 - D)$$

$$2\frac{dH}{dt} = 2b(pq - H) \tag{2.4.4}$$

$$\frac{dR}{dt} = b(q^2 - R)$$

{see Ex. 2.6}. It follows that

$$\frac{dp}{dt} = \frac{dD}{dt} + \frac{dH}{dt} = b(p^2 - D + pq - H) = 0.$$

Therefore, as before, when there is no selection, the gene pool frequencies do not change, so we can write the solution as

$$p(t) = p(0) = D(0) + H(0).$$

Since p and q are constants, we can also solve (2.4.4):

$$
\begin{aligned}
D(t) &= p^2 + e^{-bt}(D(0) - p^2) \\
2H(t) &= 2pq + e^{-bt}(2H(0) - 2pq) \\
R(t) &= q^2 + e^{-bt}(R(0) - q^2).
\end{aligned}
$$

Therefore, we see that no matter what are the genotype frequencies initially (as long as $0 < p(0) < 1$), the population will approach Hardy–Weinberg proportions at an exponential rate that is determined by the birth rate.

These results can be plotted using DeFinetti's diagrams as shown in Figure 2.2. We draw an equilateral triangle having altitude 1, and label the vertices **aa**, **ab**, and **bb** starting from the lower left and proceeding counter-clockwise. Points in the triangle can be located using triangular coordinates $(D, 2H, R)$, where D is the distance to the point from the side opposite **aa**, $2H$ is the distance from the side opposite **ab** and R is the distance from the side opposite **bb**. It follows that $D + 2H + R = 1$. This is called DeFinetti's diagram since he used triangular coordinates to describe genetic traits.

Let us draw the triangle just described and on it the locus of points $(p^2, 2p(1 - p), (1 - p)^2)$ as the parameter p ranges from 0 to 1.0 as shown in Figure 2.2A {Ex. 2.5}. The locus of the points parametrized by p is called the Hardy–Weinberg equilibrium set.

In the case of no selection, the population begins at the point $(D(0), 2H(0), R(0))$ and moves vertically on the line $D + H = p(0)$ toward the Hardy–Weinberg equilibrium set.

Slow Selection: Consider the case where the birth and death rates of the various genotypes are almost equal, say

$$b_j = b + \epsilon B_j \quad \text{and} \quad d_j = d + \epsilon D_j$$

for $j = 1, 2, 3$, where ϵ is a small scaling number. Then

$$\frac{dD}{dt} = b(p^2 - D) + \epsilon(B_1\, p\, D + B_2\, p\, H - D_1\, D - \overline{M}\, D)$$

$$2\frac{dH}{dt} = b(2pq - 2H) + \epsilon((B_3\, R + B_2\, H)p + (B_1\, D + B_2\, H)q - D_2 2H - \overline{M}\, 2H)$$

$$\frac{dR}{dt} = b(q^2 - R) + \epsilon(B_3\, q\, R + B_2\, p\, H - D_3\, R - \overline{M}\, R)$$

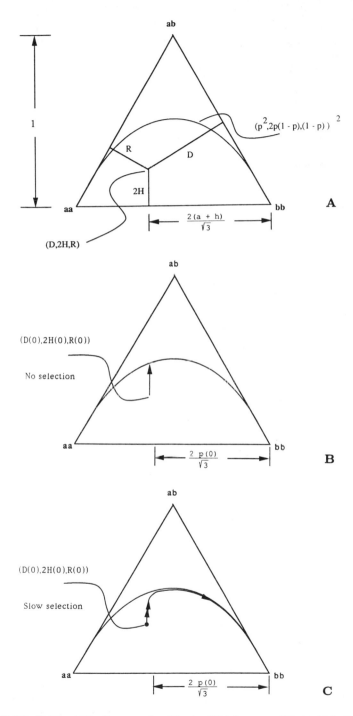

FIGURE 2.2. DeFinetti's diagram for Hardy–Weinberg equilibria (**A**), for the case of no selection (**B**), and for the case of slow selection (**C**).

where $m = b - d + \epsilon M$. We could substitute $p = D + H$, etc., into this system, but the equations are neater as written. Now,

$$(D, 2H, R) \rightarrow (p, 2pq, q) + O(\epsilon) \quad \text{as} \ \ t \rightarrow \infty$$

but p is no longer constant.

Therefore, in the slow selection case, the population distribution will approach to within $O(\epsilon)$ of the Hardy–Weinberg proportions. Now, note that if the population is close to Hardy–Weinberg proportions, then the equation for p becomes (to leading order in ϵ)

$$\frac{dp}{dt} = \epsilon\, p(1 - p)((\rho - 2\sigma + \tau)p + \sigma - \tau) \tag{2.4.5}$$

where we have set

$$\rho = B_1/2 - D_1, \ \sigma = B_2/2 - D_2 \ \text{and} \ \ \tau = B_3/2 - D_3.$$

With this, we see that formula (2.4.1) is justified if selection is slower than reproduction. (Recall that Hardy–Weinberg proportions, which were needed for this calculation, are approached at rate b, the birth rate. Hence, our assumption of slow selection is that it is slow relative to reproduction time.) The result is illustrated in Figure 2.2C where it is shown that the population distribution quickly approaches the Hardy–Weinberg equilibrium set, after which it moves slowly (since $dp/dt \sim \epsilon$) as determined by Equation (2.4.5). The factor ϵ appears in this equation because the time scale on which selection acts is ϵt whereas in Equation (2.4.1) we used h as an increment of selection time.

General selection. Hardy–Weinberg proportions are not necessarily relevant in the general case. For example, the proportions $D = \frac{1}{3}, 2H = \frac{1}{3}$, and $R = \frac{1}{3}$, for which $DR \neq H^2$, are maintained if all of the birth rates are equal, say to b, and if $d_2 = 3b/4$ but $d_1 = d_3 = 0$. This is an extreme form of disruptive selection since H is strongly selected against. In fact, the equilibrium is unstable but if the population starts there it does not approach Hardy–Weinberg proportions. Under a wide variety of conditions, Hardy–Weinberg proportions are not observable in solutions {Ex. 2.9}.

2.5   Summary

The study of genetics in this chapter began with a derivation of a difference equation to model the gene pool changes in a synchronized population. That model accounted for selection, and it gives a good and simple picture of the process.

Next, we considered the effects of small population sampling on genetics. When the population is small, random sampling of the parents' gene pool to construct the next generation can lead to the loss of a gene from the population. We saw this in two cases, one an important application in biotechnology, namely the plasmid stability problem, and the other in small human populations. The model of randomness, the Markov chain model, in each case has no randomness in it, but it is rather a model of the probabilities of various outcomes of sampling. This important step enables us to predict the distribution that should be observed in a population after many generations, and serves as the basis for statistical analysis of sampling from small populations. We will go further with the analysis of Markov chain models in the next two chapters using computer simulations and mathematical analysis.

Hardy–Weinberg proportions are observed in many field experiments using electrophoretic tests of real populations. Our analysis of Hardy–Weinberg proportions involves some lengthy calculations with models for overlapping generations, but for the genotype frequencies rather than the gene pool frequencies. By modeling the genotypes, we understand the role that the Hardy–Weinberg proportions play. Namely, we see that the Hardy–Weinberg proportions are approached if there is slow selection (relative to the birth rate). Once near these proportions, the population moves slowly as though guided by selection alone. In general, Hardy–Weinberg proportions are not to be expected.

Present work in population biology is focused on many locus–many allele genetic traits accounting for mutations and assortative matings. The models become quite complicated in these cases, but they can be managed and they have produced useful insights {Ex. 2.10}. Molecular genetics is work in a different direction. In particular, the attempt is being made by many laboratories to obtain the DNA sequence of entire chromosomes. There is much successful activity in this area, but the issues of population genetics remain [5].

In this chapter we have encountered for the first time models of random behavior. We also derived a nonrandom model for the same system. We will also see in Chapters 3 and 4 that there are important and useful connections between these two approaches to modeling, but ones that are not obvious from the beginning. In rough terms, the random sampling effects are important in small populations (fewer than 30), but usually become less important in large populations. The nonrandom model predicts certain aspects of random genetic drift, but in the sense of some specialized mean value as we will see in Chapter 3. Markov chain models are about the easiest introduction to dynamics in noisy systems. They are usually easy to derive, but often difficult to "solve," as we will also see in the next two chapters

2.6   Annotated References

1. H.F. Judson, *The eighth day of creation*, Simon and Shuster, New York, 1979.

   An interesting review of how the science of genetics developed and is used.

2. J.F. Crow, and M.Kimura, *An introduction to population genetics*, Harper & Row, New York, 1970.

   A useful resource in population genetics.

3. W. Feller, *An introduction to the theory of probability and its applications*, J. Wiley-Interscience, New York, 1966.

   One of the most important texts in probability. It is a reliable reference for the random sampling processes discussed here.

4. R. Novick, and F. C. Hoppensteadt, *On plasmid incompatibility*, Plasmid, **1** (1978) 421–434.

Exercises

2.1. SELECTIVE PRESSURE IN THE GENE POOL

Consider the model (2.1.2) for the dynamics of the gene pool determined by a one-locus, two-allele trait. Describe the behavior of g_n in the following cases: $R = S = T; R > S > T; R > S, T > S; S > R, S > T; R = S > T; R = S, T = 0$.

2.2. PLASMID CURE RATES

A simple assay used by plasmid biologists counts the number of cells that have both plasmid types for two resistant strains at each generation. This gives the rate at which cells are "cured," that is, the rate at which immunity to both antibiotics is lost from the population when it is in nonselective media.

   The cure rate can be determined theoretically by using certain properties of the transition probability matrix P. Namely, we iterate P a number of times, and call the result P^n. The norm of this matrix is denoted by $| P^n |$. Then cure rate $\sim | P^{n+1} - P^n | / | P^n - P^{n-1} |$ (n large).

   Show that for the data in Table 2.2 the cure rate is 0.86.

2.3. FISHER–WRIGHT CHAIN SIMULATION

Using a hand calculator, simulate the Fisher–Wright chain in Section 2.3 with $N = 2$ and $p_1^{(0)} = 1$. Present the answer in tabular form as in Table 2.2.

2.4. GENE POOL DYNAMICS: INFINITESIMAL SAMPLING

We saw in Section 2.1 that the gene pool proportions each generation, say g_n, are determined by the recursion formula

$$g_{n+1} = (\rho \, g_n^2 + \sigma \, g_n(1 - g_n))/w_n$$

where $w_n = \rho \, g_n^2 + 2 \, \sigma \, g_n(1 - g_n) + \tau(1 - g_n)^2$.

   If we consider the same problem when there are infinitesimal sampling intervals, then we consider a function $p(t)$ such that for some small step size, say h, $p(nh) = g_n$.

   Suppose that $\rho = 1 + \alpha h, \sigma = 1 + \beta h$, and $\tau = 1 + \gamma h$. Show that

$$dp/dt = p(1 - p)((\alpha - 2\beta + \gamma)p - \alpha + \beta).$$

This is the equation describing the continuous time analog of the model gene pool.

   Under what conditions on the fitnesses will there be a stable polymorphism? That is, a stable equilibrium for this equation where $0 < p(\infty) < 1$. This ensures that both alleles are permanently established in the population.

2.5. DeFinetti Diagram.

DeFinetti used triangular coordinates for plotting simultaneously the three genotype proportions $(D, 2H, R)$ as described in Section 2.4. Let D denote the proportion of the population being type **aa**, $2H$ the proportion of type **ab**, and R the proportion of type **bb** that are determined by a single-locus, two-allele trait. Then $D + 2H + R = 1$.

Draw an equilateral triangle having altitude 1. Label the vertices **aa**, **ab**, and **bb** starting from the lower left and proceeding counter-clockwise. Points in the triangle can be located using triangular coordinates (u, v, w) where u is the distance to the point from the side opposite **aa**, v is the distance from the side opposite **ab**, and w is the distance from the side opposite **bb**. Show that $u + v + w = 1$ for such a point.

Draw the locus of points $(p^2, 2p(1 - p), (1 - p)^2)$ as the parameter p ranges from 0 to 1. Show that this is a parabola. The locus of these points is called the Hardy–Weinberg equilibrium set. Draw the straight line $u + v = 1$ on this graph. Where does it cross the line between **aa** and **bb**?

Describe the dynamics of the genotype frequencies in the four cases of **a** dominant, **b** dominant, heterosis and disruptive selection, and plot your answers on DeFinetti's diagram as in Figure 2.2.

2.6. Genotype Frequencies

Derive the Equations (2.4.2) for D, $2H$, and R from the equations for $x, 2y$, and z.

2.7. Hardy–Weinberg Equilibria

Show that $H^2 = DR$ if and only if the population is in Hardy–Weinberg proportions (that is, reproduce the argument given in the text). The difference $H^2 - DR$ measures the distance of a population from Hardy–Weinberg proportions. Plot this function over DeFinetti's triangle. Where are maxima and minima? If $D(t), 2H(t)$, and $R(t)$ are solutions of the equations you derived in 2.6, then calculate

$$\frac{d}{dt}(H^2 - DR).$$

2.8*. Markov Chain Analysis

A Markov chain is defined by its transition probabilities $P_{i,j} =$ Prob {the process moves from state i to state j} and the state probabilities $p_{i,n} =$ Prob {the process is in state i at sampling time n}. The state probabilities at the next sampling will be

$$p_{j,n+1} = \sum_{i=1}^{M} p_{i,n} P_{i,j}$$

for $j = 1, ..., M$, the number of possible states. Setting $\mathbf{P} = (P_{i,j})$ and $\mathbf{p}_n = (p_{1,n}, ..., p_{M,n})$, we can describe this change by the vector equation

$$\mathbf{p}_{n+1} = \mathbf{p}_n \mathbf{P}.$$

Therefore, back-substitutions gives

$$\mathbf{p}_n = \mathbf{p}_0 \mathbf{P}^n.$$

This exercise enables us to evaluate this formula.

The matrix P can be written in its spectral decomposition

$$\mathbf{P} = \sum_{j=1}^{M} \lambda_j \mathbf{P}_j$$

where λ_j is the jth eigenvalue of $\mathbf{P}$, and $\mathbf{P}_j$ is a projection matrix. That is, for each j the equation $\mathbf{p}\,\mathbf{P} = \lambda_j\,\mathbf{p}$ has a nonzero solution for $\mathbf{p}$ and for each $i \neq j, \mathbf{P}_i\,\mathbf{P}_j = 0$, but $\mathbf{P}_i\,\mathbf{P}_i = \mathbf{P}_i$.

Show that

$$\mathbf{P}^n = \sum_{j=1}^{M} \lambda_j^n \mathbf{P}_j.$$

All of the eigenvalues of $\mathbf{P}$ satisfy $|\lambda| \leq 1$. Suppose that the eigenvalues $\lambda_1 = ... = \lambda_k = 1$ and the remaining eigenvalues satisfy $|\lambda_j| < 1$ for $j = k+1, ..., M$.

Therefore, show $\mathbf{p}_n \to \mathbf{p}_0(\mathbf{P}_1 + ... + \mathbf{P}_k)$ so this simple formula gives the final distribution of the process among the possible states.

Apply this result to the Fisher–Wright chain for $N = 5$. What is the population's distribution after 10 generations?

2.9* SELECTION

Using a computer, solve the system of equations you derived in 2.6 for D, $2H$, and R, assuming that $d = 0$ in each of the following four cases:

Case	b_1	b_2	b_3	$D(0)$	$2H(0)$	$R(0)$
1	1.1	1.0	0.9	0.45	0.1	0.45
2	0.9	1.0	1.1	0.45	0.1	0.45
3	0.9	1.0	0.9	0.45	0.1	0.45
4	1.0	1.0	0.9	0.45	0.1	0.45

Plot your answers on DeFinetti diagrams in each case.

2.10*. A ONE-LOCUS, THREE-ALLELE TRAIT

Consider a one locus, three allele trait having alleles **a**, **b**, and **c**. Now the gene pool has three parts, and so can be modeled using the frequencies p, q, and r where p is the proportion of the gene pool that is of type **a**, q that of type **b**, and r that of type **c**. Derive a model for how these frequencies change with time, say p_n, q_n, r_n.

Derive a corresponding model for the case of overlapping generations.

Solve the problem in the cases where there is slow selection and plot you answer (p, q, r) using triangular coordinates. (Note that $p + q + r = 1$.)

3

A Theory of Epidemics

The spread of a contagious disease involves interactions of two populations: the susceptibles and the infectives. In some diseases these two populations are from different species. For example, malaria is not passed directly between animals but by the anopheline mosquitoes, and schistosomiasis is passed from animal to animal only through contact with water in which live snails that can incubate the disease-causing helminths. In other diseases, the infection can be passed directly from infectives to susceptibles: Viral diseases like chicken-pox, measles, and influenza, and bacterial diseases like tuberculosis can pass through a population much like a flame through fuel. In this chapter, we consider diseases that propagate by direct contact.

There are useful analogies between epidemics and chemical reactions. A theory of epidemics was derived by W.O. Kermack, a chemist, and A.G. McKendrick, a physician, who worked at the Royal College of Surgeons in Edinburgh between 1900 and 1930. They introduced and used many novel mathematical ideas in studies of populations [1]. One important result of theirs is that an infection determines a threshold size for the susceptible population, above which an epidemic will propagate. Their theoretical epidemic threshold is observed in practice, and it measures to what extent a real population is vulnerable to spread of an epidemic. At roughly the same time, V.I. Semenov [2] derived a theory of combustion that identified explosion limits beyond which combinations of pressure and temperature cause chemicals to begin explosive chain-branched reactions. The two calculations are quite similar. Thresholds of population size beyond which there might be an epidemic are derived and discussed in this chapter.

The propagation of infection is modeled to determine what aspects of a population might be controlled to reduce the risk of an epidemic. We begin with the Reed–Frost model, which describes the spread of infection in populations due to random sampling. The second model is due to Kermack and McKendrick. It is a nonrandom model that describes propagation in large populations. The connections between these models are described in the second section, and a calculus-based version of the Kermack–McKendrick model is derived and solved in the third section.

These models can serve as building blocks to study other diseases, for example ones having intermediate hosts, and diseases in stratified populations, for example where there are mixing groups that have various contact probabilities, like families, preschools, schools, and social groups. Some of these extensions are described in the exercises.

3.1 Spread of Infection Within a Family

What happens when an infectious disease is introduced into a small family? What is the likelihood of spread within the family? We can answer these questions by carefully counting the possibilities.

Consider a fixed population and assume that three kinds of individuals in it are defined by a disease: susceptibles, infectives, and removals. Susceptibles can acquire the infection upon effective contact with an infective, infectives have the disease and are capable of transmitting it, and removals are those who have passed through the disease process but are no longer susceptible or infective. The flow of the disease is described by the graph

$$S \to I \to R$$

indicating that susceptibles might become infectives, and infectives might be removed, but there is no supply of new susceptibles to the process, etc.

There are problems with taking such a simple view of a disease. For example, there are great variations in the level of susceptibility, infectiousness, and immunity among individuals in populations. Also, these definitions may depend on stratifying attributes such as age groups, genetic type or mixing groups, etc. There are many diseases whose transmission mechanisms are not known, nor how long are latency periods between becoming infective and the appearance of symptoms.

Despite all of these limitations, we proceed to model the spread of a simple disease. The population is monitored at fixed sampling times, and the numbers in these classes at the nth sampling time are labeled S_n, I_n and R_n, respectively. The population is assumed to be constant during the course of the disease with size N so

$$S_n + I_n + R_n = N.$$

The population is also assumed to be randomly mixing, so that each individual has equal probability to make effective contact with any other one. Let p denote the probability of effective contact between any susceptible and any infective during one sampling interval. Finally, we suppose that the sampling intervals are exactly the same length as the duration of infectiousness in infectives. We will do away with this assumption later. At the end of the nth sampling interval, the population is examined and new numbers S_{n+1}, I_{n+1}, and R_{n+1} are observed and recorded.

The probability that a susceptible avoids contact with all I_n of the infectives during the sampling interval is

$$q_n = (1 - p)^{I_n}.$$

Therefore, the probability that $S_{n+1} = k$ is

$$\binom{S_n}{k} q_n^k (1 - q_n)^{S_n - k}$$

TABLE 3.1. Disease in a Family of Five: The First Two Weeks ($S_0 = 4$, $I_0 = 1$, $p = .05$, Period of Infection is Two Weeks)

	Observation S_1,	I_1,	R_1	Probability of this Observation
a	4	0	1	$Pr[S_1 = 4, I_1 = 0] = 0.81$
b	3	1	1	$Pr[S_1 = 3, I_1 = 1] = 0.17$
c	2	2	1	$Pr[S_1 = 2, I_1 = 2] = 0.01$
d	1	3	1	$Pr[S_1 = 1, I_1 = 3] = 0.005$
e	0	4	1	$Pr[S_1 = 0, I_1 = 4] = 0.005$

which is a simple *binomial distribution*. That is, the probability that k survive the sampling interval as susceptibles is the number of ways k can be selected from among S_n candidates times the probability that k avoid effective contact and the probability that $S_n - k$ have effective contact. If $S_{n+1} = k$, then $I_{n+1} = S_n - k$ and $R_{n+1} = R_n + I_n$.

This calculation is summarized by the formula

$$Pr[S_{n+1} = k \mid S_n \text{ and } I_n] = \binom{S_n}{k} q_n^k (1 - q_n)^{S_n - k} \qquad (3.1.1)$$

and this is called the *Reed–Frost* model [3]. This is a Markov chain model, but it is more complicated than the ones studied in Chapter 2 since the probability q_n depends on I_n and so changes from one sampling time to the next.

It is not possible to solve the Reed–Frost model, but some experiments using a hand calculator give indications of how a disease propagates.

For example, suppose that $S_0 = 4$, $I_0 = 1$, and $p = .05$. Table 3.1 shows the probabilities of various outcomes at the first sampling time. From Table 3.1 we see that it is most likely that the infection will die out without recruiting any new infectives, but there is a small chance (probability $= .005$) that all susceptibles will become infective during this first interval.

One possible evolution of the disease can be simulated using these probabilities. First, plot the probabilities in Table 3.1 on an unit interval as shown in Figure 3.1. Next, draw a random number either by rolling a die and dividing the value by the number of faces on it or by using a random number generator on a calculator or a computer. Plot the number. It will fall within one of the five intervals, and so select the letter of that interval as the outcome of the experiment. For example, the number might be 0.96, so interval b is hit and

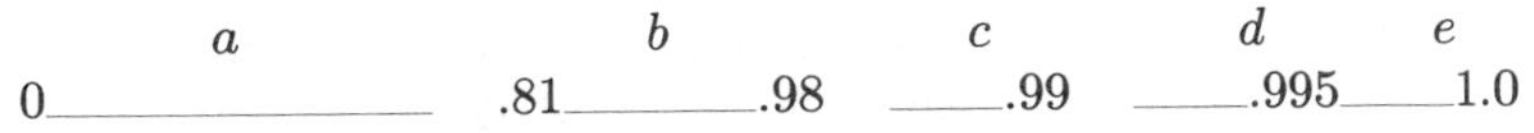

FIGURE 3.1. Probability intervals for the data in Table 3.1.

TABLE 3.2. Disease in a Family of Five after Two Periods ($S_1 = 3, I_1 = 1$)

	Observation $S_2,$	$I_2,$	R_2	Probability of this Observation
a	3	0	2	$Pr[S_2 = 3, I_2 = 0] = 0.86$
b	2	1	2	$Pr[S_2 = 2, I_2 = 1] = 0.135$
c	1	2	2	$Pr[S_2 = 1, I_2 = 2] = 0.005$
d	0	3	2	$Pr[S_2 = 0, I_2 = 3] = 0.000$

TABLE 3.3. Disease in a Family of Five after Three Periods ($S_2 = 2, I_2 = 1$)

	Observation $S_3,$	$I_3,$	R_3	Probability of this Observation
a	2	0	3	$Pr[S_3 = 2, I_3 = 0] = 0.90$
b	1	1	3	$Pr[S_3 = 1, I_3 = 1] = 0.095$
c	0	2	3	$Pr[S_3 = 0, I_3 = 2] = 0.005$

we say that

$$S_1 = 3 \quad \text{and} \quad I_1 = 1.$$

The process can be repeated: First, we recalculate the probabilities of possible outcomes as shown in Table 3.2. Again we split the unit interval into subintervals corresponding to these probabilities —now there are four intervals. Suppose that we draw 0.9. This will fall in interval b, so we have

$$S_2 = 2 \quad \text{and} \quad I_2 = 1.$$

Table 3.3 shows the possibilities if we begin with these values. In this experiment we draw 0.25 (interval a), so the infection has died out of the family after infecting three while two survived the 6 weeks in which the infection was present {see Ex. 3.1}.

We have just constructed a sample path of the process by this simulation. In real simulations, at each step a random number is drawn first and then the lengths of the intervals $a, b, \ldots$, are calculated until the random number is hit. This saves computation of all probabilities in most cases.

It is interesting to repeat the sample path simulation many times and then calculate statistics of the results using the collection of sample paths. We could calculate the average duration of the disease in a family, the expected number of people infected, etc. To illustrate this, we consider a disease in a family of five under three different assumptions about its infectiousness.

We consider the Reed–Frost model in three cases, $p = .1$, $p = .3$, and $p = .5$. In each case, we repeat the simulation, like in Tables 3.1 through 3.3, 40 times. That is, we consider the spread in 40 identical families as predicted by the Reed–Frost model. We will score the infection's success in each case by determining the number of susceptibles who have not been infected at the time when the infection disappears from the population. We call this S_∞ to indicate that it is the ultimate value of this number, although in fact the disease always drops out in no longer than five steps. $S_\infty = 2$ in the simulation in Table 3.3 {Ex. 3.1}.

The results of these simulations are presented in Table 3.4.

TABLE 3.4. Final Size for 40 Sample Paths of the Reed–Frost Model for each of Three Choices for p.

S_∞	$p = .1$	$p = .3$	$p = .5$
0	1	12	23
1	1	8	12
2	5	3	1
3	11	3	1
4	22	14	3
	—	—	—
	40	40	40

When $p = .1$, one of the 40 simulations resulted with no surviving susceptibles ($S_\infty = 0$), but 24 resulted in no further infectives appearing. When $p = .5$, 23 of the simulations resulted in all becoming infectives ($S_\infty = 0$). This table can be constructed in less than an hour using a hand calculator, or much more quickly, even using many more iterations than 40, using a programmable calculator or a computer {see Ex. 3.2}.

Table 3.4 illustrates several important points. When the disease is highly infectious ($p = .5$), there are three cases where an epidemic did not run. However, in 23 cases there are no survivors. In the case of low infectiousness ($p = .1$), only two sample paths result in severe epidemics where $S_\infty = 0$ or 1.

Note that as p increases, the distribution of survivors changes. It moves from one whose mode (highest frequency cell) is at $S_\infty = 4 (p = .1)$ to one having two modes ($S_\infty = 0$ and $S_\infty = 4$) to one that has a single mode at $S_\infty = 0$. In all cases there are some simulations where the infection dies out without recruiting any new infectives. This becomes unlikely as p increases, but it is as likely as a severe epidemic in the middle case. Is $p = .3$ near a threshold value beyond which an epidemic will propagate? It is difficult to answer this question directly from the Reed–Frost model.

Simulations of this kind have been important in planning immunization scheduling in large populations, as was done for polio vaccines. Also, they provide the only practical way for discovering the behavior of Markov chains that are as complicated as the Reed–Frost model.

As the population becomes large, we can turn away from the random model and get similar useful information about thresholds from a nonrandom model.

3.2   The Threshold of an Epidemic

In order to avoid confusion with the notation used in the the preceding section, where the variables S_n, I_n, and R_n denote random variables whose distributions were prescribed by the Reed–Frost model, we let x_n denote the number of susceptibles, y_n the number of infectives, and z_n the number of removals. These numbers will change according to the Kermack–McKendrick model that we derive next.

It might be expected that the number of susceptibles in the next sampling interval would be

$$x_{n+1} = (1 - p)^{y_n} x_n \qquad (3.2.1)$$

since the factor $(1 - p)^{y_n}$ is the proportion of susceptibles who avoid effective contact with all infectives. In fact, this is the expected value of S_{n+1} given $S_n = x_n$ and $I_n = y_n$. However, this formula does not tell how the expected values of the susceptibles $E[S_n]$ evolve. In fact, those numbers are given by the formulas

$$E[S_{n+1} \mid S_n, I_n] = (1 - p)^{I_n} S_n,$$

but they involve I_n in a nonlinear way at each step. So the connection between $E[S_{n+1}]$ and $E[S_n]$ does not follow from this formula. We will compare the implications of the model (3.2.1) with the results obtained from the Reed–Frost model (3.1.1) to understand how the two models are related.

Let $a = -\log(1 - p)$ so that e^{-a} is the probability that a given susceptible will successfully avoid contact with each infective during the sampling interval. We will now let go of the assumption that the sampling interval is the same as the interval of infectiousness. Suppose that those leaving the susceptible class enter directly into the infectious class, and that a proportion, say b, of the infectives remain infective at the end of each sampling interval. Then

$$
\begin{aligned}
x_{n+1} &= e^{-a y_n} x_n \\
y_{n+1} &= (1 - e^{-a y_n}) x_n + b\, y_n
\end{aligned}
\qquad (3.2.2)
$$

We do not keep track of the removals since the formula

$$z_{n+1} = z_n + (1 - b) y_n$$

determines their numbers, and they play no further role in the disease process. The model (3.2.2) is the *Kermack–McKendrick* model [1,4].

Will an infective more than replace itself? Let us look at the first step assuming that $y_o = 1$:

$$y_1 - 1 = b - 1 + (1 - e^{-a}) x_0.$$

This is positive if

$$x_o > (1 - b)/(1 - e^{-a}) \equiv x^*. \qquad (3.2.3)$$

If the susceptible population size exceeds the critical number x^*, then an epidemic will propagate since the infectives gain new recruits. The number

$1 - b$ is the probability of an infective not surviving to the next sampling period. Improved scrutiny and treatment of the population by public health officers can increase this number. The number $1 - e^{-a}$ is the probability of being infected. This can be decreased by reducing contacts between individuals, for example by quarantine {Ex. 3.3}.

Formula (3.2.3) gives x^* as being the threshold value of the population. It gives a useful criterion for controlling a disease. We can increase the threshold level in either of the two ways just discussed or we can reduce the susceptible population below x^*. All of these techniques have been used in various disease outbreaks over time. Of course, the best solution to epidemics would be its eradication or at least the discovery of cures for the disease.

Table 3.5 presents the results of three simulations using the Kermack–McKendrick model. These are for a large threshold, an intermediate threshold and a small threshold.

The numbers x_{∞} and y_{∞} denote the (approximate) limit values of x_n and y_n as $n \to \infty$. In the first case, the infectives never replace themselves, and the disease does not propagate. In the second case, most of the susceptible population is eventually infected, so a severe epidemic takes place over five sampling intervals. Note that some susceptibles survived the outbreak. In the last case, a short and intense outbreak occurs with all of the susceptible population being infected within three sampling intervals {see Ex. 3.4}.

The simulations in Table 3.5 can be related to the ones in Table 3.4 by observing that if we scale the susceptible and infective populations, then the value of a scales by the inverse factor since the model for $u_n = x_n/5$ and $v_n = y_n/5$ is

$$
\begin{aligned}
u_{n+1} &= e^{-5av_n} u_n \\
v_{n+1} &= (1 - e^{-5av_n}) u_n + b\, v_n.
\end{aligned}
$$

In the three cases in Table 3.5, a = 0.02, 0.07, and 0.149, respectively. Evaluating the formula $p = 1 - e^{-5a}$ in each case gives 0.1, 0.3, and 0.5, respectively, which are the values used in Table 3.4. As in Table 3.4, the first and third cases resulted in no epidemic and a severe one, respectively, and an epidemic that left some survivors resulted in the second case. The value x_{∞} for the Kermack–McKendrick model gives the approximate value of the Reed–Frost mode of S_{∞} corresponding to the epidemics that *do* propagate [see **5**]. Although x_{∞} does not give the expected value of S_{∞} in each case, it does indicate the size of most of the epidemics that do run.

3.3   Calculation of the Severity of an Epidemic

If an epidemic runs, how severe will it be? That is, what will x_{∞} be? Although this calculation can be carried out directly for the model (3.2.2), it is interesting to consider the case of infinitesimal sampling intervals to take advantage of calculus. Suppose that there are smooth functions $S(t)$, $I(t)$, and

TABLE 3.5. Solutions of the Kermack–McKendrick Model in Three Cases: $(b = 0, x_0 = 25,$ and $y_0 = 5$ in each Case)

1. $a = 0.02$. The threshold population size is $x^* \sim 50$.

Sampling Interval n	x_n	y_n
0	25	5
1	22.6	2.379
2	21.6	1.051
3	21.1	0.4
∞	$x_\infty = 20.9$	$y_\infty = 0$

2. $a = 0.07$. The threshold population size is $x^* \sim 15$.

Sampling Interval n	x_n	y_n
0	25	5
1	17.6	7.4
2	10.5	7.1
3	6.4	4.1
4	4.8	1.6
5	4.3	0.5
∞	$x_\infty = 4.1$	$y_\infty = 0$

3. $a = 0.149$. The threshold population size is $x^* \sim 10$.

Sampling Interval n	x_n	y_n
0	25	5
1	11.9	13.1
2	1.7	10.2
3	0.4	1.3
∞	$x_\infty = 0.3$	$y_\infty = 0$

$R(t)$ and a small sampling interval h such that $x_n = S(nh), y_n = I(nh)$, and $z_n = R(nh)$. Since the sampling interval h is small, we must rescale a and b: Let $a = rh$ and $b = 1 - h\sigma$. Then setting $t = nh$, we have

$$\begin{aligned}
S(t+h) &= e^{-rhI(t)}S(t) \\
I(t+h) &= (1 - h\sigma)I(t) + (1 - e^{-rhI(t)})S(t) \\
R(t+h) &= R(t) + (1 - (1 - h\sigma))I(t).
\end{aligned}$$

It follows that

$$\begin{aligned}
S(t+h) - S(t) &= (\exp(-rhI(t)) - 1)S(t) \sim -rhI(t)S(t) \\
I(t+h) - I(t) &= -h\,\sigma\,I(t) + (1 - \exp(-rhI(t)))S(t) \\
&\sim -h\,\sigma\,I(t) + rhI(t)S(t) \\
R(t+h) - R(t) &= h\,\sigma\,I(t).
\end{aligned}$$

Dividing these equations by h and passing to the limit $h = 0$ gives three differential equations for approximations to $S(t)$, $I(t)$, and $R(t)$; which we write as

$$\frac{dS}{dt} = -r\,I\,S$$

$$\frac{dI}{dt} = r\,I\,S - \sigma\,I \tag{3.3.1}$$

$$\frac{dR}{dt} = \sigma\,I$$

This system of equations is the continuous-time version of Kermack and McK-endrick's model (3.2.2). Incidentally, the calculation just completed gives a neat derivation of the *law of mass action* in chemistry in which the rate at which two chemical species, say having concentrations S and I, interact is proportional to the product SI. Thus, the law of mass action follows from the binomial distribution of random interactions since the expected number of interactions occurring in a specified (short) time interval is

$$(1 - q_n)S_n = (1 - \exp(-rhI_n))S_n \sim rhI_nS_n.$$

Obviously, this law and the two models derived for epidemics depend on the assumption that the populations are thoroughly mixing as the process continues {Ex. 3.6}.

We can solve the differential equations and so determine the severity of an epidemic. Taking the ratio of the first two equations gives

$$\frac{dS}{dI} = -\frac{r\,I\,S}{r\,I\,S - \sigma\,I} = \frac{-r\,S}{r\,S - \sigma}.$$

Therefore,

$$dI = \left(\frac{\sigma}{rS} - 1\right)dS.$$

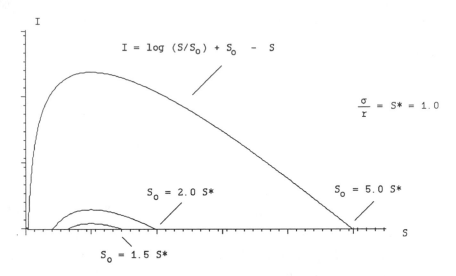

FIGURE 3.2. I versus S in two cases: $S_o > S^*$ and $S_o \gg S^*$.

Integrating this equation gives

$$I = (\sigma/r)\log S - S + C$$

where C is a constant of integration that is determined by the initial conditions:

$$C = I_o - (\sigma/r)\log S_o + S_o.$$

Typical trajectories are shown in Figure 3.2

In the infinitesimal sampling process, the threshold level of S^* becomes

$$S^* = (1 - b)/(1 - e^a) \sim \sigma/r.$$

S^* is the value of S for which $dI/dt = 0$. We see in Figure 3.2 that trajectories starting near but above this value describe epidemics that end at a comparable distance below this value. Trajectories that start well above S^* end up near $S = 0$. However, in each case the final size of the susceptible population, $S(\infty)$, is where the trajectory meets the $I = 0$ axis. Therefore, solving the equation

$$S - (\sigma/r)\log S = C$$

for its smaller of two roots gives the final size. This is not possible to do in a convenient form; however, it is easy to do using a computer. In this way, we can estimate an epidemic's severity once we have estimated the infectiousness (a or r) and the removal rate (b or σ) {see Ex. 3.7}.

Recurrent diseases. Finally, there are diseases in which removals can eventually become susceptible again. This is the case for a variety of sexually transmitted diseases, for example gonorrhea. The flow of such a disease is depicted by the graph

$$S \to I \to S.$$

Without further discussion, we can write down a model of such a disease:

$$dS/dt = -rIS + \sigma I$$
$$dI/dt = rIS - \sigma I.$$

Since $I + S$ is constant (its derivative is zero), we can reduce these equations to a single equation

$$dS/dt = (\sigma - rS)(I_o + S_o - S).$$

We see that if $S^* = \sigma/r < I_o + S_o$, then $S \to S^*$ in this case! In the other case, $S \to I_o + S_o$, and the infection dies out of the population. When $S \to S^*$, the disease is endemic {Ex. 3.11}.

Stratification of the population, latency periods of the disease, hidden carriers, seasonal cycling of contact rates, and many other factors confound the study of epidemics, but the simple models derived here provide useful and interesting methods.

3.4 Summary

The study of epidemics, although often gruesome, is quite interesting and important. For example, why is it that when an epidemic goes through a school, there are some who survive as susceptibles? The calculation of the epidemic threshold shows how this can happen. If S_0 is near or below the threshold S^*, then few or no susceptibles will become infective because there is not enough effective contact or the infectives are removed quickly enough. So there is a kind of "herd immunity." New diseases imported to a highly susceptible population, that is, one much greater than S^* for the disease, can devastate a population as smallpox did in Central America and AIDS is doing to subpopulations around the world now. In other cases, isolated populations can be driven to a carrying capacity S^* that is limited not by nutrients but by a local disease. When new susceptibles immigrate, the population can be rapidly pushed above S^*, and the ensuing epidemic will reduce the total population to a level below S^*, by a number comparable to the size of the immigration. Reproduction will eventually move the population up toward the threshold level even though there might be a reservoir of disease.

Epidemics have been modeled using the Reed–Frost and Kermack–McKendrick models. We have seen that the Reed–Frost model is based on a Markov chain that can be described using simulations [3]. The simulation method used here is called the Monte Carlo method [6], and it is widely used to study random processes that have not been "solved" using other methods. The construction of sample paths gives a better understanding of how random processes can propagate. Propagation of rumors and the behavior of crowds have been studied using models like the Reed–Frost and Kermack–McKendrick models [4]. Recent work on AIDS and other diseases [7], [8], [9] has been carried out using various extensions of these basic models {Exs. 3.8, 3.9, 3.10, 3.11}.

3.5   Annotated References

1. W. O. Kermack, and A.G. McKendrick, *A contribution to the theory of epidemics*, Proc. Roy. Soc.(A) **115** (1927), 700-721, **139** (1932), 55–83.

   Classic papers in the theory of epidemics. See also A.G. McKendrick, *Mathematics applied to medical problems*, Roy. Soc. Edinb., 1926.

2. N. N. Semenov, *Chemical kinetics and chain reactions*, Oxford Univ. Press, Oxford, 1935.

3. N.T.J. Bailey, *The theory of infectious diseases and its applications*, Charles Griffin, London, 1975.

   An excellent resource for epidemic modeling.

4. F. C. Hoppensteadt, *Mathematical methods of population biology*, Cambridge Univ. Press, 1982.

5. D. Ludwig, *Stochastic population theories. Lect. Notes Biomath*, vol 3, Springer–Verlag, New York, 1974.

   A good account of and introduction to stochastic differential equations used in population models.

6. J.M.Hammersley, and D.C. Handscombe, *Monte Carlo methods*, Methuen, London, 1964.

   An excellent introduction to computer simulation of random processes.

7. J.M. Hyman, and E.A. Stanley, *The effect of social mixing patterns on the spread of AIDS, Lect. Notes Biomath*, vol 81 (Chavez, Levin, Shoemaker, eds.), Springer-Verlag, New York, 1989, 190-219.

8. R.M. May, and R.M. Anderson, *Transmission dynamics of HIV infections*, Nature **326** (1987), 37–42.

9. J.A. Yorke, and W. London, *Recurrent outbreaks of measles, chickenpox and mumps*, Am. J. Epidemiol. I(98) (1973), 453–468; II(98) (1973), 469–482.

Exercises

3.1. REED–FROST SIMULATION IN A FAMILY

Carry out the Reed–Frost simulation as described in Tables 3.1 through 3.3.

3.2. FINAL SIZE OF REED–FROST EPIDEMICS

Reproduce the results in Table 3.4 by carrying out the Reed–Frost simulation described there.

3.3. KERMACK-MCKENDRICK THRESHOLD

Consider the sequence x_n, y_n that is generated by the Kermack–McKendrick model (3.2.2) with $z_0 = 0$.

a. Show that the following limit exists:

$$x_\infty = \lim_{n \to \infty} x_n.$$

b. Show that

$$\lim_{n \to \infty} y_n = 0.$$

(Hint: Use the first equation in (3.2.2).) Deduce that $z_\infty = N - x_\infty$.

c. Show that $x_n = x_0 \exp(-az_n/(1-b))$.

d. Let $F = x_\infty/x_0$. F measures the final size of the susceptible population and $1 - F$ is the severity of the epidemic. Show that

$$F = \exp\left(-\frac{ax_0}{1-b}\left(1 + \frac{y_0}{x_0} - F\right)\right).$$

e. Let $T = ax_0/(1-b)$ and $y_0/x_0 = i = 0.01$. Solve the equation in d. for F for values of $T, 0 \le T \le 3.0$ by steps of 0.01 using Newton's method. Plot your answers by plotting F vs. T.

f. Explain what happens at $T = 1$.

3.4. FINAL SIZE OF KERMACK–MCKENDRICK EPIDEMICS

Reproduce the results in Table 3.5.

3.5 ASYMPTOMATIC CARRIERS

Consider a population in which there are infectives who cannot be detected. We denote their numbers of C. In that case, the Kermack–McKendrick model becomes

$$x_{n+1} = x_n e^{-a(y_n+C)}$$

where C gives the number of these carriers. Describe what happens to the solution in this case.

3.6. THE LAW OF MASS ACTION

Begin with the binomial distribution and derive the law of mass action. In particular, $E[S_1 - S \mid S, I] = S(1-p)^I - S$. Show that if p is near 0, then this is (approximately) proportional to IS.

3.7. SOLUTIONS OF THE KERMACK–MCKENDRICK MODEL

We obtained the equation $I = (\sigma/r) \log S - S + C$ by solving system (3.3.1). Set $I = 0$ and solve for S using Newton's method. Plot your results as a function of rS_o/σ. Compare this result to the one you obtained in Exercise 3.3 using F.

3.8. EPIDEMICS WITH INTERMEDIATE CLASSES

Some diseases place new recruits from the susceptible class into an "exposed, but not yet infectious" class, which we denote by E. The graph $S \to E \to I \to R$ describes the process.

   a. Derive a mathematical model for this disease using either difference equations or differential equations. Consider two cases:

      i. A certain proportion of the exposed group becomes infective at each sampling time $(dE/dt = -r_o E)$.

      ii. Individuals remain in the exposed class for a fixed time, say T $(dE/dt = r_o I(t)S(t) - r_o I(t-T)S(t-T))$.

   b. Derive a threshold result for this system in either of the cases in part a.

3.9*. SPREAD OF AN INFECTION IN TWO SMALL FAMILIES

Formulate a Reed–Frost model for the spread of a disease within and between two identical families of five each. Assume that there is a different contact rate between families than within them. Simulate the spread of an infection in the combined group beginning in one family. Estimate the severity of the epidemic and present your results in tabular form as in Table 3.4.

3.10*. SCHISTOSOMIASIS

Schistosomiasis is a disease caused by a wormlike parasite (a helminth). Male and female helminths must mate in a host (e.g., humans, ducks, or swine). Thereafter, some of the fertilized eggs leave the host in its feces. When an egg comes in contact with fresh water, it hatches and attempts to find a snail that it can penetrate. Once a snail is infected, a large number of larvae are produced. They swim freely in search of a host in which to reproduce. It might penetrate the skin of a host or be ingested with water or food grown in the water. We sample the populations at regular intervals, and we denote by H_n the mean number of worms infecting each host, I_n is the number of infected snails. Then

$$H_{n+1} = (1 - \mu)H_n + c\, I_n$$
$$I_{n+1} = (1 - \delta)I_n + b\frac{(S - I_n)H_n^2}{1 + H_n}$$

where μ and δ are death probabilities of hosts and snails, c is the number of helminths becoming established in a host due to each infected snail, S is the number of snails (fixed) and the term $bH_n^2/(1 + H_n)$ gives the mean number of paired worms per infected host and so is proportional to the number of eggs produced. The last term describes the interaction between eggs and susceptible snails.

Consider the steady state distributions of helminths and infected snails: $H_n = H$ and $I_n = I$. The equations for these values are

$$H = (1 - \mu)H + c\, I$$
$$I = (1 - \delta)I + b\frac{(S - I)H^2}{1 + H}.$$

a. Describe the static states of the schistosomiasis model.

b. Which of these solutions are stable?

3.11*. RECURRENT DISEASES: RELAPSE–RECOVERY MODEL

Relapse–recovery diseases are denoted by the graph

$$S \to I \to S.$$

Suppose that after a fixed length of time, say τ, an infective returns to being fully susceptible again. Then instead of the model in Section 3.3, we have

$$\frac{dS}{dt} = -r\, I(t)S(t) + r\, I(t - \tau)S(t - \tau)$$
$$\frac{dI}{dt} = -r\, I(t - \tau)S(t - \tau) + r\, I(t)S(t).$$

Since $I + S = N$, we have the single equation

$$dI/dt = r(I(t)(N - I(t)) - I(t - \tau)(N - I(t - \tau))).$$

a. It is known that $I \to I^*$, a constant, as $t \to \infty$. Determine the value of I^*.

b. Test the stability of I^*.

4

Biogeography

Bacteria in our guts, insects in a field, trees in a forest and plants borne by air and water around the world are among many examples whose spatial distributions are important and interesting to study. Mechanisms of dispersal include making small random moves, being carried along by air or water, and being attracted to certain areas by chemical signals, nutrients, light, etc. Patterns of organisms can be formed by dispersal or aggregation. On the other hand, immobile organisms, like some bacteria on plant roots, can find themselves in habitats where nutrition fluctuates, for example by nutrients being washed through the soil in regular cycles. Patterns of organisms can also be formed by uneven distribution of nutrients or toxins.

The patterns of organisms that result from these forces can be important in how they influence their environment or how they survive adversity. For example, there are foci of infectious diseases in human populations [1] and foci of infestation insects in forests [2] that cause recurring outbreaks. If these could be identified, then eradication might be possible. In another case, patterns of bacterial growth in habitats having gradients of nutrients, antibiotics or mutagens are used as diagnostic tools in medicine and as engineering tools in biotechnology [3]. In addition, the geographic distributions of blood types in humans have provided useful data for anthropologists and historians: These distributions are records of major events like migrations or long periods of isolation [4].

Biogeography deals with the spatial distribution of organisms, and in this chapter we study three problems of biogeography. First, foci of activity are described in two separate settings using cellular automata. Next, we use random walk models to study how distributions can change due to migration of organisms. Finally, we consider growth of fixed populations subjected to an environment through which diffuses a nutrient.

Many of the ideas in the preceding chapters can be applied to understanding aspects of biogeography. We begin with the Game of Life and some extensions of it that indicate how data of spatial distributions can be generated and how the processes work. Next, we study how random walks are related to these problems, and how they can be traced and applied. The result is a Markov chain model. Finally, we derive a calculus-based model, based on the diffusion equation, that enables us to derive more useful information from the random walk model.

An important element in mathematical modeling is presented in this chapter. We have seen how random phenomena can sometimes be described using

Markov chains; for instance, the evolution of genetic traits or the spread of an infection were modeled in Chapters 2 and 3 using vectors of probabilities of the various possible outcomes and a matrix of probabilities of possible changes between outcomes over each sampling interval. These discrete-time models can be studied using computer simulations, but it is usually difficult to "solve" them. Of course, the word "solution" has various meanings to various people. For example, a computer simulation might be exactly what is needed to interpret or design an experiment. On the other hand, if one would determine how sensitive or robust a phenomenon is to changes in environmental parameters, a formula that shows explicitly how the solution depends on the parameters would be desirable.

Most random processes are closely related to normal distributions. This important fact was established by statisticians, and the result is usually summarized in a central limit theorem that shows how to scale random variables to relate them to a normal distribution [5]. Once a connection has been established between a problem and normal distributions, many useful statistical methods can be applied to estimate parameters and to establish confidence intervals. Although we do not go into this statistical theory here, we do derive an important connection between random walk Markov chains and normal distributions. In particular, we show in this chapter that the random-walk Markov chain can be approximated by a differential equation, the diffusion equation, whose solutions are normal distributions. Similar approaches can be used to study the genetics problems described in Chapter 2 and the epidemics in Chapter 3.

4.1   The Game of Life

A topographical map can be divided into small segments and the counts of an organism inhabiting each segment can be recorded. The numbers might be placed at the midpoint of each segment and updated at regular sampling-time intervals. The result is a sequence of maps that describes the dynamic changes of the population's spatial distribution—like a motion picture where each frame is one of the updated maps. It is possible to describe both these spatial and temporal movements as the solution of a mathematical model that involves both space and time variables.

The Game of Life is an idealized version of this, and it nicely illustrates the underlying ideas. The game was introduced by J. Conway in a *Scientific American* article in 1970 [6], and it has captured the interest of mathematicians and computer students.

We consider a grid on the plane labeled by integer pairs. For example, the site (i, j) is located at the point in the plane having integer coordinates i units horizontal from the origin and j vertical. We denote by $S_{n,i,j}$ the number of organisms observed at site (i, j) at the nth sampling time. Resolution as fine as the number of organisms might not be needed, or even possible, and the only information collected might be a score if a site is occupied or vacant at

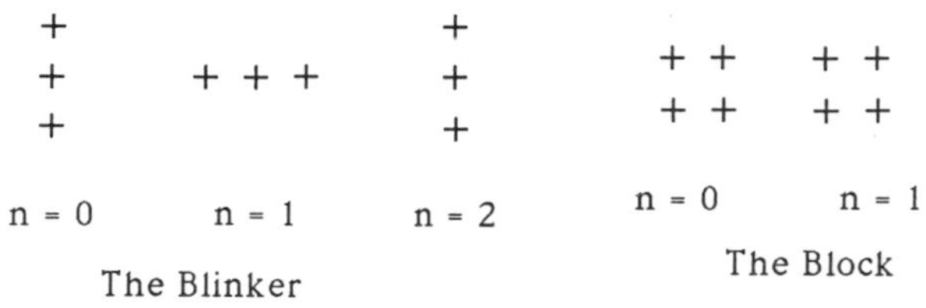

```
+                    +
+      + + +         +        + +    + +
+                    +        + +    + +
+                    +

n = 0    n = 1     n = 2      n = 0       n = 1

     The Blinker                  The Block
```

FIGURE 4.1. Here + denotes $S = 1$ and blank indicates $S = 0$. The blinker pattern goes on oscillating between the two configurations shown, but the block pattern is a stable configuration that does not change {see Ex. 4.1}.

each sampling. For example, we could write $S_{n,i,j} = 1$ if site (i,j) is occupied and $S_{n,i,j} = 0$ otherwise.

We consider the latter case. In the Game of Life these numbers will change at each tick of a timing clock according to the following rules:

1. An occupied site having two or three neighboring sites occupied will continue to be occupied. (There are *eight* neighbors to each site.)

2. Each occupied site having no, one, or four or more occupied neighbors becomes vacant.

3. Each vacant site becomes occupied if it has exactly three occupied neighbors.

Figure 4.1 gives two examples of how these rules work.

The Game of Life model is an example of a *cellular automaton*, that is, a spatial array of cells whose contents change with time according to some specific rules.

Another interesting cellular automaton was introduced by Norbert Wiener in 1947 [7]. It allows there to be more states at each site than just two. We now consider a distribution of sites, each having three possible states. To fix ideas, we use the analogy of a forest infested with defoliating insects. The three possible states of a site are green, infested with defoliating insects, or defoliated. These states are indicated, respectively, by $S = 0$, $S = 1$, and $S = -1$, and the following rules describe their dynamics. In each sampling period

1. an infested site becomes defoliated $(1 \rightarrow -1)$

2. a defoliated site becomes green $(-1 \rightarrow 0)$

3. a green site becomes infested if any of its four nearest neighbors is infested $(0 \rightarrow 1$ if so).

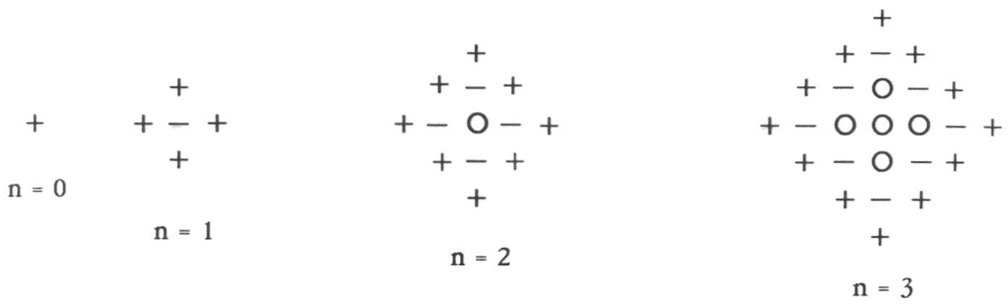

```
                                                      +
                                                    + − +
                            +                     + − O − +
              +           + − +         + − O − +   + − O O O − +
  +         + − +       + − O − +       + − O − +   + − O − +
            +           + − +             + − +
  n = 0                  +                 +
            n = 1                          +
                         n = 2
                                           n = 3
```

FIGURE 4.2. A wave of infestation propagating outward from a single infestation.

The model is illustrated in Figure 4.2, where it is shown that a single infested site generates a wave of infestation propagating outward, followed by a wave of defoliation.

There are possible foci of infestation that reproduce themselves and so maintain the infestation. Two are shown in Figures 4.3A and 4.3B.

The reader might like to show that if a habitat is seeded with a period three focus and elsewhere with a period four focus, then eventually the habitat becomes synchronized with period three {See Ex. 4.2}.

Now consider the same system distributed over the surface of a sphere. Suppose each site represents a muscle cell that is at rest (0), contracting (1), or in a refractory state (-1) after contraction. If the same rules for changing the state of sites are used, then a single contracting cell at one pole of the sphere will cause a wave of contraction to spread uniformly around the sphere to the antipode. The refractory wave that follows the wave of contraction will quench activity at the antipode, and the array will return to rest. If at the pole there is a periodic array, like in Figure 4.3, then regular waves of contraction will be created and they will propagate to the antipode in a regular progression, roughly similar to heart contraction.

These models can be made more realistic by assuming that it takes many sampling intervals for a refractory site to become resting again, etc., but it is already a difficult model to study. For example, it is difficult to find foci of activity in an established pattern. This and problems like it remain unsolved for this model.

A further extension of this approach involves plotting actual numbers at each grid point that quantify the level of activity at the site. For example, suppose that a thin layer of bacteria has been spread over the surface of an agar pour plate. If the agar contains all needed nutrients save one, then the cells cannot grow. However, if a drop of the missing nutrient is placed at the center of the plate, some cells there will begin growing. As the drop spreads out, more growth will be observed. How fast will a drop spread out? What will the growth pattern be at various sampling times? These questions will be discussed later. Such an experiment, called the Ames test [3], is used for testing mutagenicity of carcinogens. In that, a plate of *Salmonella typhimurium* that are growing on minimal growth media is tested by placing a drop of the

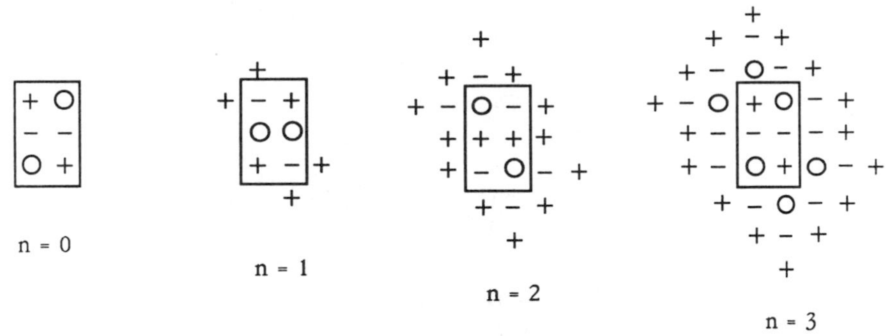

```
 +----+            +            +  -  +              +
 |+ O |        +  | - + |   +  - +          +  -  O  -  +
 |- - |        + | O O |      +  -| O  -|+       +  -  O | + O | -  +
 |O + |        + | + - | +     + | + + |+      +  -| -  - |-  +
 +----+            +        +  | -  O | -  +     +  -| O + |O  -  +
  n = 0            +            +  -  +          +  -  O  -  +
               n = 1           +                   +  -  +
                             n = 2                    +
                                                   n = 3
```

FIGURE 4.3A. Platt's three-period focus [8]. The rectangular area keeps track of the original focus. It is reproduced after three time steps.

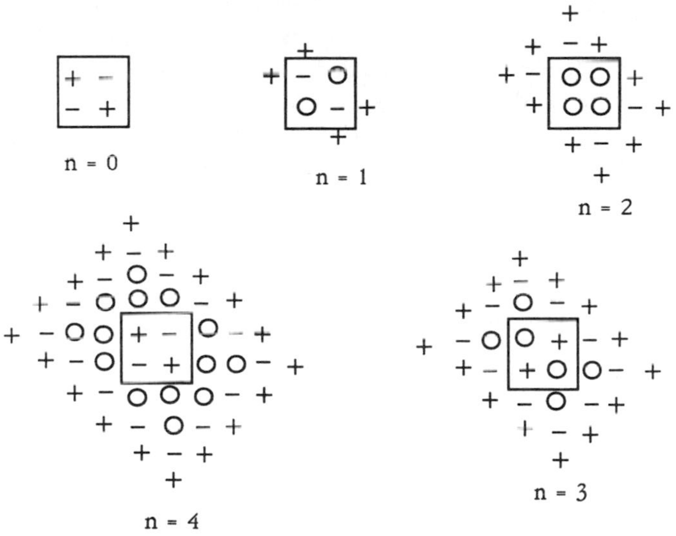

```
  +----+            +              +  -  +
  |+ - |       +  | - O |     +  -| O O |+
  |- + |       + | O - |+     + | O O |-  +
  +----+            +              +  -  +
   n = 0        n = 1                +
                                  n = 2
```

```
         +                         +
      +  -  +                    +  -  +
   +  - O -  +                +  -  O  -  +
+  - O O O -  +           +  - O| O +|-  +
+  - O|+ -|O  -  +        +  -| + O|O -  +
+  - O|- +|O O -  +        +  -  O  -  +
   +  - O O O -  +          +  -  +
      +  - O -  +              +
      +  -  +               n = 3
         +
      n = 4
```

FIGURE 4.3B. A four-period focus. In both cases, regular waves of infestation are generated that propagate outward. The wavelength is three in Figure 4.3A, and it is four in Figure 4.3B.

carcinogenic growth factor at the center and scoring the genetic changes that occur in population as the drop spreads.

4.2   Random Walks

The Game of Life and the variants mentioned in the preceding section are nonrandom, that is, once the initial distribution of the states is given, there is only one possible evolution of the system. It is interesting and useful to study the effect of small random fluctuations in a dispersal system and to derive as a result an overarching but manageable model.

Consider now a long line of trees, for example along a river. Some are infested with an insect, like a fruit fly. We count the number of insects in each tree and we attempt to describe how these numbers change by formulating rules that are consistent with our observations of the insect's behavior.

First, a labeling of the trees is needed. We pick one tree, called 0, to set a frame of reference, and locate trees from that site, say m is the mth tree to the right and $-m$ is the mth tree to the left. The proportion of insects in the mth tree at the nth sampling is denoted by

U_{mn} = proportion of the total population that is in tree m at sampling time n.

The basic assumptions are:

1. The insects are counted at fixed sampling time intervals.

2. In each sampling interval, an insect will move to the nearest tree on the left with probability $q(q < 1/2)$, to the tree on the right with probability q, and it will remain in its present tree with probability $1-2q$. q measures the mobility of the insects, and the term "probability of movement" refers to the fact that if a large number of insects are in a tree now, then a proportion q of them move left, q right and $1 - 2q$ remain fixed.

We are ignoring the wind, habitat preference, and many other features in making this assumption. Also, we suppose that there is no reproduction or death during the interval we are counting, so the total population remains constant through our experiment.

Insects moving according to these rules are said to be executing a *random walk*. These rules are sufficient to enable us to derive a useful mathematical model: The number in the mth tree at sampling time $n + 1$ will be the proportion that remain there from the previous time plus those that immigrate from adjacent trees. This is described in Equation (4.2.1).

$$U_{m,n+1} = q\, U_{m+1,n} + q\, U_{m-1,n} + (1 - 2q)U_{m,n} \qquad (4.2.1)$$

This model is capable of providing an accurate qualitative description of the infestation. It shows how the numbers change in time along the line of trees, and it is illustrated in Table 4.1.

TABLE 4.1. Random Walk with $q = 0.05$

n	$m = -3$	$m = -2$	$m = -1$	$m = 0$	$m = 1$	$m = 2$	$m = 3$
0				1			
1			0.05	0.9	0.05		
2		0.0025	0.09	0.815	0.09	0.0025	
3	0.0001	0.0068	0.1229	0.7425	0.1229	0.0068	0.0001

Suppose now that the line of trees in not unlimited, but extends from tree $-M$ to tree M. There are three important and manageable ways of treating what happens at the end trees. They are called *boundary conditions*, because they indicate what happens at the ends of the domain we are studying.

Periodic boundary conditions. Suppose that the line of trees surrounds a lake, so the trees M and $-M$ are neighbors. In this case we replace where needed U_{M+1} in the equations by U_{-M} and U_{-M-1} by U_M.

Absorbing boundary conditions. In this case, the trees are in a line, but the two end trees are controlled so that $U_{-M} = 0$ and $U_M = 0$. Insects who move into these end trees just disappear.

Reflecting boundaries. For this, we place an imaginary tree next to each of the end trees and define $U_{-M-1} = U_{-M+1}$ and $U_{M+1} = U_{M-1}$. The result is that

$$U_{-M,n+1} = 2qU_{-M+1,n} + (1 - 2q)U_{-M,n}$$

and

$$U_{M,n+1} = 2qU_{M-1,n} + (1 - 2q)U_{M-1,n}$$

but the rest of the formulas are the same as before.

All three of these boundary conditions arise naturally in the study of various random processes [5] {see Ex. 4.3}.

Since we have normalized the counts in each tree by the total population size,

$$\sum_{m=-M}^{M} U_{m,n} = 1$$

In fact, we can consider the vector $\mathbf{p}_n = (U_{-M,n}, U_{-M+1,n}, \dots, U_{M,n})$ to be a probability vector that describes the probability distribution of the insects among the trees.

In the case of periodic boundary conditions, we have that

$$\mathbf{p}_{n+1} = \mathbf{p}_n \begin{pmatrix} 1-2q & q & 0 & 0 & 0 & q \\ q & 1-2q & q & 0 & 0 & 0 \\ 0 & q & 1-2q & 0 & 0 & 0 \\ & \vdots & & \ddots & \vdots & \\ 0 & 0 & 0 & 1-2q & q & 0 \\ 0 & 0 & 0 & q & 1-2q & q \\ q & 0 & 0 & 0 & q & 1-2q \end{pmatrix}.$$

The matrix of probabilities of possible changes reflects the periodic boundary conditions in this case. This model is referred to as a random walk Markov chain on a circle. Note that each row of this matrix and each column of the matrix add up to 1. Such a matrix is called a *doubly stochastic matrix*. It is possible to derive useful results from this matrix, but as simple as it appears, it still presents difficulties for analysis. Similar formulations can be made for the cases of reflecting and absorbing boundaries and for the unlimited domain {Ex. 4.8}.

Direct computer simulation of these models is quite straightforward, and there are quite useful matrix methods for solving them in other ways as well [see **5**].

4.3   The Diffusion Approximation

The random-walk model can be converted into a differential equation that can be solved. Suppose that there are many trees and that they are closely packed. A continuous labeling of sites is convenient now, so let x range from -1 to +1, where $x = m/M$ is the location of the mth tree. We write $\delta x = 1/M$ and view M as being very large. Also, suppose that the sampling time intervals are short, and let t denote the time variable and δt the length of a sampling interval. We will try to find a smooth function $u(x, t)$ such that

$$u(m\,\delta x, n\,\delta t) \sim U_{m,n}$$

where δx and δt are small numbers.

Substituting this into the random walk model (ignoring boundary conditions, if there are any) gives

$$u(x, t + \delta t) = q\,u(x + \delta x, t) + q\,u(x - \delta x, t) + (1 - 2q)u(x, t).$$

Rearranging this equation and dividing both sides by δt and δx^2 gives

$$\frac{u(x, t + \delta t) - u(x, t)}{\delta t} = q\frac{\delta x^2}{\delta t}\frac{u(x + \delta x, t) + u(x - \delta x, t) - 2u(x, t)}{\delta x^2}.$$

The mathematical trick here, that was uncovered by Albert Einstein [**9**], is to let δx and δt approach zero in such a way that $q\delta x^2/\delta t =$ constant, say D. Then the equation for u becomes

$$\frac{\partial u}{\partial t} = D\frac{\partial^2 u}{\partial x^2}. \tag{4.2.2}$$

This is referred to as the *diffusion equation* and the coefficient D is called the *diffusivity*. D is closely related to the *variance* of the random walk since it is proportional to q. This equation arises in many descriptions of biological and physical phenomena, including *Brownian motion* [**9**], gradient driven chemical diffusion (*Fick's law*), and heat flow [**10**] {see Exs. 4.4, 4.5}. The equation plays a crucial role in probability theory and statistics. In fact, a diffusion equation can be associated with each Markov chain, as we modeled the random walk with one, and in that way important properties of the chain can be uncovered.

The four problems we described earlier translate into the following problems for the diffusion equation:

Unlimited domain. When $-\infty < x < \infty$, an important solution has the form

$$u(x,t) = \frac{\exp\left(-\frac{x^2}{4Dt}\right)}{\sqrt{4\pi Dt}}.$$

(The reader should verify that this is a solution of the diffusion equation.) The graph of this function is a bell-shaped curve of a normal distribution having a variance $(2\pi Dt)$ that increases with time. The whole realm of ideas involving Markov chains, diffusion approximations, the central limit theorem, which states that most random processes suitably scaled are very close to normal distributions, and the law of large numbers, is fascinating [see **5**].

Periodic boundary conditions. The formulas

$$u(-1,t) = u(1,t) \quad \text{and} \quad (\partial u/\partial x)(-1,t) = (\partial u/\partial x)(1,t)$$

force u to have period 2 in x.

Absorbing boundaries. The formulas

$$u(-1,t) = 0, u(1,t) = 0$$

describe the absorbing boundary case.

Reflecting boundaries. The conditions

$$\frac{\partial u}{\partial x}(-1,t) = 0, \frac{\partial u}{\partial x}(1,t) = 0$$

describe reflecting boundary conditions.

In the reflecting and periodic cases the solution must approach a constant as $t \to \infty$. The solution in the absorbing case must approach zero as $t \to \infty$ {see Ex. 4.10}.

Unfortunately, simple closed form solutions are not known in the cases of limited domains, although the solutions can be constructed using Green's functions, Fourier series, or Laplace transforms [**11**].

Let us return to the unlimited domain case. A number of interesting things can be determined about diffusions without too much technical work. A solution to the diffusion equation is

$$u(x,t) = \frac{\exp\left(-\frac{x^2}{4Dt}\right)}{\sqrt{4\pi Dt}}.$$

This function has been normalized with the coefficient $1/\sqrt{(4\pi Dt)}$ so that the total area under its graph is 1. Because of this property and the fact that function is nonnegative, we say that it is a *probability distribution*, like the vector distributions that we have been working with, except that it is indexed by a continuous variable x. The distribution that this function describes is for a random variable x, and the probability of finding x in an interval $a < x < b$ is given by the integral

$$\int_a^b \frac{\exp\left(-\frac{x^2}{4Dt}\right)}{\sqrt{4\pi Dt}}\,dx.$$

As $t \to 0$, the function $u(x,t)$ gets very large at $x = 0$, reflecting that all of the "probability" is focused closer and closer to $x = 0$. To be precise, the limit as $t \to 0^+$ is the Dirac delta function! This only makes sense when we interpret this function $u(x,t)$ using integrals: As $t \to 0^+$, we say that the distribution $u(x,t)$ approaches $\delta(x)$, Dirac's delta function, because the limit of this integral is 1 for any interval $a < x < b$ that contains $x = 0$, and is zero otherwise. Therefore, the solution $u(x,t)$ describes the diffusion of a substance that is initially concentrated at $x = 0$.

4.4   The Growth of Bacteria on Plates

We can repeat this entire calculation for habitats that cover a two-dimensional region, say in the xy-plane. By deriving the random-walk model and assuming that $\delta x^2/\delta t \to D$ and $\delta y^2/\delta t \to D$ as before, we obtain a diffusion approximation in two spatial dimensions that is described by the equation

$$\frac{\partial u}{\partial t} = D\left(\frac{\partial^2 u}{\partial x^2} + \frac{\partial^2 u}{\partial y^2}\right)$$

{see Exs. 4.6, 4.9}.

The two-dimensional diffusion equation can be studied in a variety of interesting ways. Usually, the domain of interest has a special geometry that suggests using an appropriate coordinate system that facilitates solving the problem. For example, to study the radially symmetric case of a drop of nutrient placed in the center of a circular petri dish filled with agar, we can describe the concentration of chemical at location (x, y) at time t by u. Since the domain and the drop are radially symmetric, we look for a radially symmetric solution by converting to polar coordinates ($r^2 = x^2 + y^2, \theta = \tan^{-1}(y/x)$). "Radially symmetric" means that we seek a solution that does not depend on θ. The diffusion equation in this case is

$$\frac{\partial u}{\partial t} = D\frac{1}{r}\frac{\partial}{\partial r}\left(r\frac{\partial u}{\partial r}\right).$$

A probability distribution solution of this equation is {See Ex 4.7}

$$u(r,t) = \frac{e^{-\frac{r^2}{4Dt}}}{4\pi Dt}.$$

We can describe the growth of cells on the plate using the Jacob–Monod model of cell growth {see Ex. 4.7}. The bacteria on the plate are fixed. If $B(r, t)$ denotes the number of cells at position r (distance from the center of the plate) at time t, then

$$\frac{dB}{dt} = \frac{\alpha A u B}{K + A u}$$

where A is the concentration of the initial drop, α is the maximum uptake rate and K is the saturation constant of nutrient whose concentration is described by $A u$. If $A u$ is near zero, there is slow growth. If $A u$ is near K, the cells are growing at half their maximum. If $A u$ is much larger than K, the cells are growing at their limiting rate α. For practical purposes, we say that the cells are growing if $A u > K$ and not if $A u < K$; that is, the saturation constant is taken as being a rough guide as to what concentration is needed for cell growth.

Using the formula for u that we found earlier, we can calculate the distance $R(t)$ from the center to where growth occurs at time t by solving the equation

$$\frac{e^{-\frac{R^2}{4Dt}}}{4\pi Dt} = \frac{K}{A}$$

for $R(t)$. The result is that the velocity of this front of growth is roughly

$$dR/dt \sim C(t \ln t)^{-1}$$

where C is a constant depending on A, K, and D. Therefore, a slowing front of growth will appear in the plate {see Ex. 4.7}. This is expected because of radial dilution of the nutrient.

We can get an idea of the rate of spread of the chemical by considering how a circle must change to keep a constant concentration outside of it. Let us attempt to find $R(t)$ such that

$$\int_0^{2\pi} \int_R^\infty u(r, t) r \, dr \, d\theta = c^*$$

where c^* is a small constant. Since $u(r, t) = \exp(-r^2/4Dt)/4\pi Dt$, we have that

$$\int_0^{2\pi} \int_R^\infty u(r, t) \, r \, dr \, d\theta = 2\pi \int_R^\infty \frac{\exp\left(-\frac{r^2}{4Dt}\right)}{4\pi Dt} r \, dr = \exp\left(-\frac{R^2}{4Dt}\right) = c^*$$

so $R^2 = 4Dt \log 1/c^*$. Typical units for D in this experiment are $\mathrm{cm}^2/\mathrm{sec}$, so the drop moves so that R^2/t is constant on a velocity scale of cm/sec. In particular, $dR/dt \sim 1/\sqrt{t}$, so the drop continues to expand, but it slows down.

4.5 * Another View of Random Walks

There is another approach to modeling random walks that sometimes clarifies the relation between random and nonrandom models. This approach is from the point of view of a sample path rather than of a total distribution of outcomes. Let us now consider the differential equation

$$dx = f(x)\, dt + \sigma\, dw$$

where $f(x)$ is a smooth function of x, σ is a constant, and dw is a random variable. We interpret this equation of differentials in the following way. A small change (dx) in x will result from a drift term $(f(x)dt)$ and some noise (σdw). The noisy increment (dw) is taken from a normal distribution having mean zero and variance 1.0. This model is called a *stochastic differential equation*. It is known that the solution of such a problem can be described in terms of a probability distribution, called $\phi(x,t)$. That is, the probability of finding x in an interval $a < x < b$ at time t would be

$$\int_a^b \phi(x,t)\, dx.$$

The equation for ϕ is

$$\frac{\partial \phi}{\partial t} = \frac{\sigma^2}{2} \frac{\partial^2 \phi}{\partial x^2} - \frac{\partial}{\partial x}(f(x)\phi).$$

This is plausible since the stochastic differential equation is like a random-walk, but with a superimposed drift f, and we have seen that the random walk model is closely related to the diffusion equation. This equation is called the Fokker–Planck equation for the distribution of positions x, in honor of two physicists who studied similar models that describe molecular motion. Note that when $f = 0$

$$\phi(x,t) = \frac{\exp\left(-\frac{x^2}{4Dt}\right)}{\sqrt{4\pi Dt}}.$$

The drift term (f) might be created by a chemical gradient that attracts population members. If $F(x)$ is the concentration of an attracting chemical signal at position x, then

$$f(x) = \frac{\partial F}{\partial x}.$$

This indicates that movement is toward increasing concentrations. The random-walk model becomes

$$dx = \frac{\partial F}{\partial x}(x)\, dt + \sigma\, dw$$

and the population distribution is found by solving the Fokker–Planck equation

$$\frac{\partial \phi}{\partial t} = \frac{\sigma^2}{2} \frac{\partial^2 \phi}{\partial x^2} - \frac{\partial}{\partial x}\left(\frac{\partial F}{\partial x}\phi\right). \tag{4.5.1}$$

A particular solution of this equation is

$$\phi(x) = C \exp\left(\frac{2F(x)}{\sigma^2}\right) \tag{4.5.2}$$

where C is a constant. The relevance of this particular solution to solving (4.5.1) is more complicated to determine [see **12**], but it does describe the population's distribution in a large habitat during certain phases of the population's movement. By plotting this solution for various values of σ, we see that

1. if σ is small, the distribution is sharply focused near the local maxima of $F(x)$

2. if σ is large, the distribution is nearly uniform

3. for intermediate values of σ, there is a balance between chemotaxis and dispersal.

These observations fit our intuition. If $\sigma = 0$, then the movement is toward maxima of F, and in the absence of the dispersal mechanism provided by the random walk, the population would accumulate at these maximum concentrations. The results suggest how the mobility of individuals (measured by σ) can interact with other forces (here chemotaxis) to create uneven distributions of a population {Ex. 4.12}.

4.6 Summary

The discussion of the diffusion approximation completes our introduction to the mathematics of populations. We have seen in the preceding chapters that population phenomena can be modeled using nonrandom difference and differential equations and random models such as Markov chains.

It is an important question is: What is the relation between the nonrandom and the random models of the same phenomenon? This is not easy to answer in all cases, but the calculations in this chapter give some insight into resolving such questions.

It is always possible to derive a corresponding nonrandom version of the random model, although care is needed in how the results are interpreted. For example, the Reed–Frost model of disease is closely related to the Kermack–McKendrick model, which describes the mean of the epidemics in the Reed–Frost model that actually do run when the population is large. But, the Kermack–McKendrick model does not estimate the probability that a disease will drop out of a population, which is possible even when it is superthreshold. If the population is small, random sampling can cause the disease to drop out in a few steps. In this case, the Kermack–McKendrick model can indicate the severity of epidemics that do run, but not the probability of the disease dropping out.

Markov chain models are attractive because they are easy to derive and to simulate on a computer. Analyzing them can be "tough as nails" since finding the eigenvalues of the probability matrix is necessary, but usually very difficult {see Ex. 2.8}. Fortunately, associated with each Markov chain is a diffusion approximation whose solution describes the probability distribution of the states of the process. Finding the diffusion approximation is often useful, but it may not always be possible. In many population problems, the variance of the random process, that is how spread out are the probabilities, is proportional to 1/population size. Therefore, the variance is reduced to near zero when large populations are considered, and it is possible to show, using stochastic differential equations, how the random models pass over into the nonrandom ones as population size increases [12]. For practical purposes, random effects in populations of size 30 or more are ignored.

There is a close connection between the theory of chemical reactions and the theory of population problems—especially epidemics, but also in biogeography. Reaction–diffusion systems in chemistry have the form

$$\frac{\partial u}{\partial t} = D\frac{\partial^2 u}{\partial x^2} + g(t, x, u)$$

where u is the concentration of a chemical, D is its diffusivity and $g(t, x, u)$ describes chemical reactions at position x at time t. Similar equations can be derived for the biogeography of genetic traits and epidemics. Analysis of such problems leads to understanding more complicated aspects of biogeography [13], [14], [15].

4.7   Annotated References

1. N.T.J. Bailey, *The theory of infectious diseases and its applications*, Charles Griffin, London, 1975.

   An excellent resource for epidemic modeling.

2. C.S. Holling, *The functional response of invertebrate predators to prey density*, Ottawa Entom. Soc. Canada, 1966.

3. P. Gerhardt, et al. *Manual of methods of general bacteriology*, Am. Soc. Microbiology, Washington, D.C., 1981.

4. A.E. Mourant, A.C. Kopec, and K. Domaniewicz-Sobczak, *The distribution of blood groups and other polymorphisms*, 2nd ed., Oxford Univ. Press, New York, 1976.

   An introduction to the use of genetics in anthropology.

5. W. Feller, *An introduction to probability theory and its applications*, vol I, J. Wiley-Interscience, New York, 1968.

   A broad, reliable and sophisticated description of probability theory.

6. J. Gardner, *Mathematical games*, Sci. Am. October (1970), 120–123.

7. J.M. Greenberg, M.B. Hassard, and S. Hastings, *Pattern formation and periodic structures in systems modeled by reaction-diffusion equations*, Bull. Amer. Math. Soc. **84** (1978), 1296–1327.

8. B. Platt, *Masters thesis*, University of Utah, 1985.

9. A. Einstein, *Investigation on the theory of Brownian movement*, Dover, New York, 1956.

   Probably the only thing in science written by Einstein that non physicists will able to understand.

10. J. Fourier, *The analytical theory of heat*, Dover, New York, 1898.

    Fourier's original and profound work on the heat equation.

11. H.S. Carslaw, and J.C. Jaeger, *Conduction of heat in solids*, 2nd ed., Oxford Univ. Press, New York, 1986.

    An excellent source for solutions of the heat equation in various geometries.

12. D. Ludwig, *Stochastic population theories*, Lect. Notes in Biomathematics, vol. 3, Springer–Verlag, New York, 1974.

13. J.D. Murray, *Mathematical biology*, Springer–Verlag, New York, 1989.

    A compendium of pattern formation models.

14. F. C. Hoppensteadt, *Mathematical methods in population biology*, Cambridge Univ. Press, Cambridge, 1982.

15. R.A. Fisher, *The genetical theory of natural selection*, Dover, New York, 1930.

Exercises

4.1. THE GAME OF LIFE

Determine the evolution of the game of life for the following initial distributions:

a.

```
+   +
+   +
+   +
+   +
```

b.

```
0   +   0
0   0   +
+   +   +
```

4.2. CELLULAR AUTOMATA

Consider the three-state model for the spread of defoliating insects in Section 4.1. Describe what happens in each of the following cases. (Determine the period of each configuration and describe the pattern generated by it.)

a.

```
0   0   0
0   +   0
0   -   0
```

b.

```
+   0   0
-   -   0
0   +   0
```

c. If a period three focus and a period four focus are started at different places of the same grid, what happens after a long time?

4.3. RANDOM WALKS

a. Use the random walk model with $q = 0.25$ and $M = 2$ to determine the evolution of the initial conditions shown in Table 4.2

Table 4.2.

Tree	-2	-1	0	1	2
# insects	0	0	100	0	0

using the reflecting, absorbing, and periodic boundary conditions in three separate simulations.

b. Construct sample paths of the random walk in part a. by using the methods in Chapter 3 for Tables 3.1 through 3.3. Present your results by listing or plotting the location of the sample individual at each sampling time. That is, construct a sample path that an individual might follow.

4.4. Diffusion Equation in an Unlimited Region

Consider the diffusion equation for $-\infty < x < \infty$

$$\frac{\partial u}{\partial t} = \frac{\partial^2 u}{\partial x^2}.$$

Show that $u(x,t) = \exp(-x^2/4t)/\sqrt{4\pi t}$ solves this equation, and that for each t, the area under this function is equal to 1.0. Because of this, we refer to u as being a probability distribution.

4.5. Statistics of the Diffusion Equation

Evaluate the mean, variance, and entropy of the distribution $u(x,t)$ in Exercise 4.4. That is, evaluate

$$\mu = \int_{-\infty}^{\infty} x\, u(x,t)\, dx$$

$$\sigma^2 = \int_{-\infty}^{\infty} (x-\mu)^2 u(x,t)\, dx$$

and

$$H = -\int_{-\infty}^{\infty} u(x,t) \log\, u(x,t)\, dx$$

respectively.

4.6. Diffusion Equation in a Two-Dimensional Region

a. Derive the diffusion equation in two dimensions (x and y) from the random walk model as shown in Section 4.4.

b. Show that

$$u = \frac{e^{-\frac{x^2+y^2}{4\pi Dt}}}{4\pi Dt}$$

solves this equation.

c. Convert both the equation and the solution to polar coordinates by setting $x = r\cos\theta$ and $y = r\sin\theta$. Verify that u solves your result.

4.7. BACTERIAL GROWTH ON A POUR PLATE

Consider the model of growth on a pour plate derived in Section 4.4. The distribution of nutrient is described by $A\, u(r,t)$, where u is given by the formula

$$u(r,t) = \frac{e^{-\frac{r^2}{4\pi Dt}}}{4\pi Dt},$$

and the bacterial population density $B(r,t)$ can be determined by solving the equation

$$\frac{dB}{dt} = \frac{\alpha A u(r,t)}{K + A u(r,t)} B(r,t).$$

Solve this problem for $B(r,t)$ by substituting the expression for $u(r,t)$ into this formula. Let $A = K/2$, $A = K$, and $A = 2K$. For each of these choices of A, plot the profile of bacteria density as a function of dish radius r at various times, say t near zero, $t = 1.0$, $t = 10.0$. How large will the region of growth be in each case? The profile you find is the record of the nutrient's movement under the bacterial population.

4.8*. STOCHASTIC MATRICES

The matrix of probabilities given in section 4.2, which we call $\mathbf{P}$ here, is for a random walk on a periodic domain. $\mathbf{P}$ is doubly stochastic; that is, the sum of each column is one and the sum of each row is one. (A matrix is called stochastic if its row sums are all equal to 1.0.) Show that the probability distribution

$$\mathbf{p}^* = \frac{1}{M+1}(1, 1, \ldots, 1)$$

is a stationary distribution for this Markov chain. That is,

$$\mathbf{p}^* = \mathbf{p}^*\mathbf{P}.$$

Conclude that 1.0 is an eigenvalue for the matrix $\mathbf{P}$. Show that all other eigenvalues satisfy $|\lambda| < 1$. Conclude that $\mathbf{p}_n \to \mathbf{p}^*$ as $n \to \infty$.

4.9*. FICK'S LAW

Consider a chemical that is in solution. Its concentration at a point (x, y, z) is denoted by $c(x, y, z, t)$. Fix a domain, say a sphere in the solution, and consider how the total mass in this domain can change. There can be creation (sources) or destruction (sinks) of the chemical, or the chemical can pass into or out of the boundary of the domain. It follows from Green's theorem in calculus that this can be represented mathematically by the formula

$$\frac{\partial c}{\partial t} - \text{ - div (Flux through the boundary)} + \text{sources - sinks}$$

Fick's Law states that the flux through the boundary that is due to diffusion is proportional to the negative gradient of c:

$$\text{Flux through the boundary} \quad = -D\,\nabla c.$$

Show that if there are no sinks or sources of material, and there is no flow of the fluid, the formula for conservation of mass is

$$\frac{\partial c}{\partial t} = D\nabla \cdot \nabla c = D\left(\frac{\partial^2 c}{\partial x^2} + \frac{\partial^2 c}{\partial y^2} + \frac{\partial^2 c}{\partial z^2}\right).$$

This gives a derivation of the diffusion equation from the point of view of mechanics. Fourier derived the heat equation, another name for the same equation, in a similar way. In that case, c represents the temperature at point (x, y, z) at time t [see **10**, **11**]. Therefore, we see that the diffusion equation arises in three separate arenas: probability theory, mechanics, and the theory of heat.

4.10*. FOURIER SERIES FOR DIFFUSION EQUATIONS WITH BOUNDARIES

If $f(x)$ is a continuously differentiable function that has period X (that is, $f(x + X) = f(x)$ for all x), then it can be written in terms of a Fourier series:

$$f(x) = \frac{a_0}{2} + \sum_{n=1}^{\infty}\left(a_n \cos\frac{2\pi nx}{X} + b_n \sin\frac{2\pi nx}{X}\right)$$

Use this fact to find Fourier series solutions of the diffusion equation in the three cases of periodic, reflecting, and absorbing boundary conditions. (Hint: Let

$$u(x, t) = \frac{a_0(t)}{2} + \sum_{n=1}^{\infty}\left(a_n(t)\cos\frac{2\pi nx}{X} + b_n(t)\sin\frac{2\pi nx}{X}\right)$$

and find equations for the unknown functions $a_n(t)$ and $b_n(t)$ in each case.) Conclude that $u(x, t) \to$ constant in the first two cases and to zero in the third.

4.11*. THE SOLUTION OF THE DIFFUSION EQUATION, GIVEN $\mathbf{u(x, 0)}$

Let $f(x)$ be a differentiable function. Show that the formula

$$u(x, t) = \frac{1}{\sqrt{4\pi Dt}}\int_{-\infty}^{\infty} \exp\left(-\frac{(x - y)^2}{4Dt}\right) f(y)\,dy$$

defines a solution of the diffusion equation by verifying that it solves the equation.

Show that

$$\lim_{t \to o^+} u(x, t) = f(x)$$

4.12*. SIMULATED ANNEALING

A formula for $\phi(x)$ was derived in Equation (4.5.2). Verify that this formula does define a solution of Equation (4.5.1). Suppose that

$$F(x) = e^{-x^2}$$

and that σ^2 is small (say 0.01), intermediate (say 0.1), and large (1.0). Plot the stationary distribution of the Fokker–Planck equation in each case. In physical applications, this process is known as annealing. In this a physical system is heated (increasing σ) and then cooled (reducing σ) to ensure that all maxima of F are occupied, and the largest maximum has the most occupants. Carry out a Monte Carlo simulation of the random walk model with drift. Do this in each of the three cases in above, and compare your results with the distribution there. (Hint:

$$x_{n+1} = x_n - 2x_n h e^{-x_n^2} + \sigma Z_n$$

where h is the step size, say 0.1, and Z_n is a normal random variable.) (Hint: At each step, a value for Z_n can be found by drawing six random variables from die tossing or a handheld calculator, adding them up, substracting their expected value—0.5–and dividing by $\sqrt{6}$.)

4.13*. A GENETIC CLINE

a. Consider a long line of sites, and at each site is located a population that carries a one-locus, two-allele genetic trait. Let $g_{m,n}$ denote the frequency of the gene pool at site m that is of type **a**. If the sites are isolated, the reproduction of the population would be described by the recursion

$$g_{m,n+1} = f(g_{m,n})$$

where $f(g) = (\rho g^2 + \sigma g(1 - g))/(\rho g^2 + 2\sigma g(1 - g) + \tau(1 - g)^2)$. We suppose that at each sampling time the population reproduces and then does a random walk to neighboring sites. Thus,

$$g_{m,n+1} = \lambda(f(g_{m+1,n}) + f(g_{m-1,n})) + (1 - 2\lambda)f(g_{m,n}).$$

Write a computer program to solve this problem for 100 sites using periodic boundary conditions. Suppose that at some sites $\rho > \sigma > \tau$ and at others $\rho < \sigma < \tau$. Using computer simulation, describe the population's final distribution of genotypes. An irregular distribution of gene pool proportions is called a *genetic cline*.

b. We showed in Exercise 2.4 that the iteration in a can be rewritten as a differential equation for the frequency of the gene pool that is of type **a**, say $p(t)$, at time t:

$$dp/dt = p(1 - p)((\alpha - 2\beta + \gamma)p - \alpha + \beta)$$

where α, β, and γ are the Malthusian fitnesses of the genotypes. Let us denote the right-hand side of this equation by $F(p)$. Then as in 2.4 we have

$$f(g) = g + hF(g).$$

i. Show that if we replace $g_{m,n}$ by a smooth function $g(x,t)$ for which $g(m\delta x, n\delta t) = g_{m,n}$ for small sampling steps and times, δx and δt, then the recursion scheme is approximated by the diffusion equation

$$\frac{\partial g}{\partial t} = D\frac{\partial^2 g}{\partial x^2} + F(g).$$

ii. If $D = 1$ and $F(g) = g(1 - g)(4 - 8g)$, then show that

$$g(x,t) = (\tanh x + 1)/2$$

is a solution of the diffusion approximation. Therefore, we have a convenient mathematical example of a cline. Explain how this cline is formed and maintained by selective pressures.

5

The Heart and Circulation

This chapter begins a discussion of mathematics in physiology to which the remainder of the book is devoted. The discussion begins with the heart and blood circulation in the body. We first outline the structure of the circulation and then we derive models of blood flow and pressure and mechanisms for controlling them.

5.1 Plan of the Circulation

The function of the heart is to pump blood. The blood carries oxygen (O_2) from the lungs to the various tissues of the body and it carries carbon dioxide (CO_2) from these tissues back to the lungs.

Since the circulation forms a closed loop, its description can begin anywhere. We will begin on the left side of the heart (see Figure 5.1). The *left heart* receives blood that is rich in O_2 and pumps this blood into the systemic arteries. These form a tree of progressively smaller vessels that supply fully oxygenated (and hence bright red!) blood to all of the organs and tissues of the body. From the smallest of the *systemic arteries*, blood flows into the systemic capillaries, which are roughly the diameter of a single red blood cell. It is in the capillaries that the actual exchange of O_2 and CO_2 takes place. The blood that leaves the systemic capillaries carries less O_2 and more CO_2 than the blood that entered. (The loss of O_2 causes a change in the color so that the blood is now more bluish than before.)

Leaving the systemic capillaries, the blood enters the *systemic veins* through which it flows in vessels of progressively increasing size toward the right side of the heart.

The *right heart* pumps blood into the *pulmonary arteries* which form a tree that distributes the blood to the tissues of the lung. The smallest branches of this tree give rise to the *pulmonary capillaries* where CO_2 leaves the blood stream and O_2 enters from the air space of the lungs. Leaving the pulmonary capillaries, the oxygenated blood is collected in the *pulmonary veins* through which it flows back to the left heart. This completes the circulation. The average time required for a red blood cell to complete the circuit that we have described is about 1 minute.

The reader has probably noticed an important symmetry in the plan of the circulation: The blood that leaves the left heart flows through the arteries, capillaries, and veins of the *systemic circulation* before returning to the

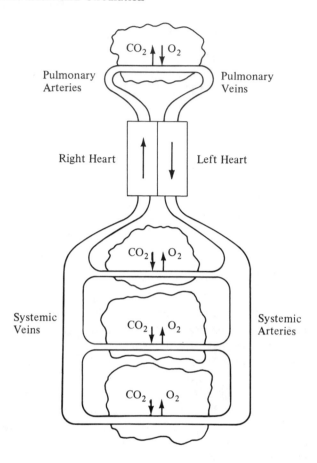

FIGURE 5.1.

TABLE 5.1. Normal Resting Pressures and Volumes of the Systemic and Pulmonary Arteries and Veins

	P(mm Hg)	V(liters)
sa	100	1.0
sv	2	3.5
pa	15	0.1
pv	5	0.4

($s =$ systemic, $p =$ pulmonary, $a =$ artery, $v =$ vein)

right heart. Similarly, the blood that leaves the right heart flows through the arteries, capillaries and veins of the *pulmonary circulation* before returning to the left heart. Of course, these partial "circulations" are not really closed loops, since there is no blood flow directly from one side of the heart to the other (except in the fetal circulation and in certain forms of congenital heart disease).

Because of this symmetry between the systemic and pulmonary circulations, we can expect that the equations of the systemic circulation will have the same form as the equations of the pulmonary circulation. Similarly, the equations of the right and left heart will be the same in form, and the relation of the right heart to the systemic circulation will be the same as the relation of the left heart to the pulmonary circulation. These symmetries in the *form* of the equations are not matched by corresponding symmetries in the *magnitude*, however. That is, the parameters appearing in the equations of the pulmonary circulation have values that are different from the corresponding parameters of the systemic circulation. Because of these differences, the systemic blood volume is about 10 times the pulmonary blood volume, and the systemic arterial pressure is about 6 times the pulmonary arterial pressure (see Table 5.1). One of the themes of this chapter is to study the consequences of this quantitative disparity between the two circulations.

5.2   Volume, Flow and Pressure

The purpose of this section is to introduce the three physical variables that are needed in a quantitative description of the circulation, to explain the system of units used by physiologists, and to give typical values that occur in the different parts of the circulation.

Since blood is nearly incompressible, the volume of the blood serves as a convenient measure of the amount of blood in any part of the circulation. Volume will be measured in *liters* (1 liter = 1000 cm^3) and designated by the symbol V. The total blood volume (V_o) is about 5 liters, partitioned roughly as shown in Table 5.1.

The definition of the *flow* that we use in this book is the volume of blood per unit time passing a point in the circulation. Thus, flow is measured in liters/minute. We designate flow by the symbol Q. The most important flow in the circulation is the *cardiac output*, which is defined as the volume of blood pumped per unit time by either side of the heart. (This definition assumes that the two sides of the heart produce identical outputs. At this point, the reader should be wondering why this is so. The mystery will be cleared up later.) The cardiac output may be calculated as the product of the stroke volume (volume of blood pumped per beat) and the heart rate (number of beats per unit time). Typical values are

$$
\begin{aligned}
\text{stroke volume} &= 70 \text{ cm}^3/\text{beat} \\
&= 0.070 \text{ liters/beat} \\
\text{heart rate} &= 80 \text{ beats/minute} \\
\text{cardiac output} &= 5.6 \text{ liters/minute}
\end{aligned}
$$

The usual definition of *pressure* (P) is force per unit area, and pressure is expressed in terms of the height of a column of mercury that can be supported by the pressure in question. (Note that this height is independent of the cross-sectional area of the column: If the area is doubled the weight of the column is doubled, but so is the force produced by a given pressure.) Thus, the conventional units of pressure in physiology are mm Hg (millimeters of mercury).

When considering pressures, it is important to remember that only pressure *differences* produce observable effects. Thus, any reference pressure can be called zero, and other pressures can be reported as differences from the reference pressure. A particularly convenient reference pressure in physiology is the pressure of atmosphere, since this is the pressure outside of most of the blood vessels of the circulation. Pressure differences with respect to the atmosphere can be measured directly by the simple device of leaving the far end of the (U-shaped) mercury column open to the atmosphere. Throughout this chapter the symbol P will stand for pressure measured with respect to the atmosphere. As we shall see, this definition of pressure has greater relevance for the circulation than the absolute pressure.

5.3   Resistance and Compliance Vessels

Consider the blood vessel shown in Figure 5.2. The volume of the vessel is V, its inflow is Q_1 at pressure P_1, and its outflow is Q_2 at pressure P_2. The external pressure is zero (atmospheric). Suppose that the vessel is in a steady state, which means that none of these quantities are changing with time. Then we must have $Q_1 = Q_2$ (why?), so we will drop the subscript and just use the symbol Q to designate either the inflow or the outflow.

How are Q, P_1, P_2 and V related? This is a complicated question since it involves two separate properties of the blood vessel: Its *resistance* to blood flow and its *compliance* in response to distending pressure. We can isolate

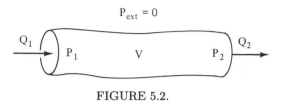

$$P_{ext} = 0$$

FIGURE 5.2.

these properties by considering special cases.

First, suppose that the tube is rigid, so that the volume is known and constant. Then we only need a relationship between Q, P_1, and P_2. Since only pressure differences matter, it is a safe assumption that Q is determined by $P_1 - P_2$. The simplest relationship of this sort is

$$Q = (1/R)(P_1 - P_2) \qquad (5.3.1)$$

where R is a constant called the *resistance* of the vessel. If a vessel satisfies (5.3.1), we call it a *resistance vessel*. Next suppose that the tube is elastic but that it has no resistance to blood flow so that the pressures at the two ends of the tube are equal for all Q. Because the tube is elastic, there is some relation between the distending pressure $P = P_1 = P_2$ and the volume V. The simplest relation of this kind is

$$V = C\,P \qquad (5.3.2)$$

where C is a constant called the compliance of the vessel.

Alternatively, if we want to take into account the nonzero residual volume of the vessel at zero pressure, we could use the relationship

$$V = V_d + C\,P \qquad (5.3.3)$$

where C is still called the compliance and where V_d is the ("dead") volume at $P = 0$. A vessel satisfying (5.3.2) or (5.3.3) is called a *compliance vessel*.

Clearly, the concepts of resistance vessels and compliance vessels are idealizations. First, a real vessel must exhibit both resistance and compliance properties simultaneously. Second, we have assumed linear relationships that may be too simple to describe real blood vessels.

The reply to these objections is as follows. First, the circulation does seem to produce a clear separation between the resistance and compliance functions of its different vessels. Thus, the large arteries and veins are primarily compliance vessels in the sense that only small pressure differences are needed to drive the cardiac output through these vessels, while their changes in volume are highly significant. The main site of resistance is in the tissues themselves (primarily at the level of the smallest arteries, the *arterioles*) where volume changes are less important but where large pressure drops are observed.

Second, the approximation of a linear relation between flow and pressure differences (5.3.1) is a good approximation when we allow for changes in resistance. This may appear to be a circular argument, since we can always make

(5.3.1) true by introducing the definition $R = (P_1 - P_2)/Q$. In fact, tissues exhibit reasonably constant values of R under conditions where the diameters of their blood vessels remain constant. When R changes, a physiological explanation must be sought. This explanation usually involves a stimulus that leads to contraction or relaxation of the smooth muscles in the walls of the arterioles. Such a stimulus may be generated by the nervous system, by circulating hormones (or other substances circulating in the blood), or by the action of locally produced products of metabolism. Some of these effects will be studied in Section 5.9 on autoregulation.

Finally, there is no such justification for the linear compliance relations that we have assumed. It is an excellent approximation to say the volume of a blood vessel is determined by the internal pressure, but the relationship between volume and pressure becomes progressively less compliant as it is distended. The linear model is introduced for simplicity.

5.4   The Heart as a Pair of Pumps

A pump is a device that can accept fluid at low pressure (P_1) and transfer it to a region where the pressure is high $(P_2 > P_1)$. Thus, the pump performs work on the fluid; the rate at which work is performed by the pump is the product of the volume rate of flow Q and the pressure difference $P_2 - P_1$. To characterize the pump we need to say how Q depends on P_1 and P_2.

Consider, for example, the left side of the heart (Figure 5.3). The left ventricle is equipped with an inflow (mitral) valve and an outflow (aortic) valve. When the ventricle is relaxed (diastole) the inflow valve is open and the outflow valve is closed. During this period of time, the left ventricle receives blood from the left atrium at a pressure that is essentially that of the pulmonary veins. Thus, for the left ventricle, $P_1 = P_{sv} = 5$ mm Hg. When the ventricle contracts (systole), the inflow valve closes and the outflow valve opens. Then the left ventricle actively pumps blood into the systemic arterial tree. Thus, for the left ventricle, $P_2 = P_{sa} = 100$ mm Hg

What determines the output of the left ventricle under these conditions? To answer this question we follow an approach introduced by Sagawa and his collaborators: We regard the ventricle as a compliance vessel whose compliance changes with time. Thus, the ventricle is described by

$$V(t) = V_d + C(t)P(t) \tag{5.4.1}$$

where $C(t)$ is a given function with the qualitative character shown in Figure 5.4. The important point is that $C(t)$ takes on a small value $C_{systole}$ when the ventricle is contracting, and a much larger value $C_{diastole}$ when the ventricle is relaxed. For simplicity, we have taken V_d to be independent of time.

Using (5.4.1), we can construct a pressure–volume diagram of the cardiac cycle (Figure 5.5). For a detailed explanation of this type of diagram, see the paper by Sagawa et al., cited in Section 5.12. For our purposes, it is sufficient

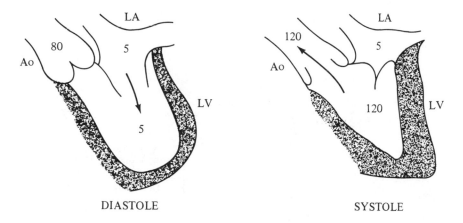

DIASTOLE   SYSTOLE

FIGURE 5.3.

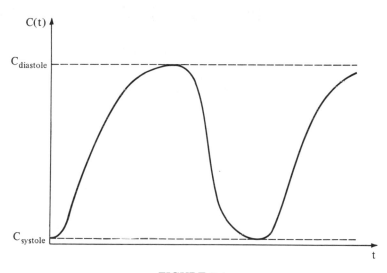

FIGURE 5.4.

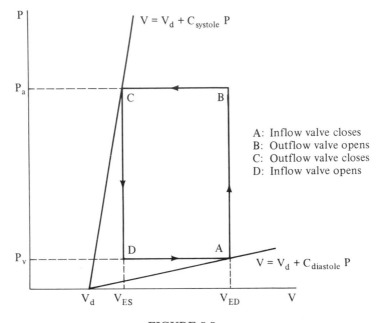

FIGURE 5.5.

to note that the maximum volume achieved by the ventricle (at end-diastole) is given by

$$V_{ED} = V_d + C_{diastole}P_v \tag{5.4.2}$$

while the minimum volume (achieved at end-systole) is given by

$$V_{ES} = V_d + C_{systole}P_a \tag{5.4.3}$$

where P_a is the pressure in the arteries supplied by the ventricle and P_v is the pressure in the veins that fill it. Thus, the stroke volume is given by

$$\begin{aligned} V_{stroke} &= V_{ED} - V_{ES} \\ &= C_{diastole}P_v - C_{systole}P_a. \end{aligned} \tag{5.4.4}$$

A particularly simple special case is when $C_{systole} = 0$, so that the systolic line is vertical in Figure 5.5. This gives a stroke volume

$$V_{stroke} = C_{diastole}P_v \tag{5.4.5}$$

which is the model of the ventricle that we shall use. Finally, if F (frequency) is the heart rate (beats per minute), we get cardiac output

$$\begin{aligned} Q &= FV_{stroke} \\ &= FC_{diastole}P_v \end{aligned} \tag{5.4.6}$$

For the present, F is taken to be constant, although we shall consider changes in heart rate later in the chapter. We define

$$K = FC_{diastole} \qquad (5.4.7)$$

so that $Q = KP_v$. We call K the *pump coefficient* of the ventricle. Although F is the same for the two sides of the heart (which are driven by the same pacemaker), the constant $C_{diastole}$ is greater in the thin-walled right ventricle than in the thick-walled left ventricle, so K is greater on the right than on the left. Also, the two sides of the heart are connected to different venous systems. Thus, we have the following expressions for the right and left cardiac outputs:

$$Q_r = K_r P_{sv} \qquad (5.4.8)$$

$$Q_L = K_L P_{pv}. \qquad (5.4.9)$$

Throughout this section we have tacitly assumed that the pressure outside the heart is zero (atmospheric). If not, then the distending pressures during diastole are not simply P_{sv} and P_{pv} but $P_{sv} - P_{thorax}$ and $P_{pv} - P_{thorax}$, where P_{thorax} is the pressure in the chest. In fact, P_{thorax} is slightly negative (with respect to the atmosphere) and this contributes to increased cardiac output by increasing the end-diastolic volume V_{ED}. This effect was first noticed because it disappears when the chest is opened during surgery. In the model developed below, we assume for simplicity that $P_{thorax} = 0$ so that we can use (5.4.8) and (5.4.9) without modification. Then, effects of $P_{thorax} < 0$ are considered briefly in Exercises 5.8 through 5.9.

5.5   Mathematical Model of the Uncontrolled Circulation

In this section, we put together the ideas that have been developed above to construct a mathematical model of the circulation. In the form that we first present it, the model lacks the control mechanisms that regulate the circulation and make it serve the needs of the body. In subsequent sections, we will use this model in several ways:

1. to study the *self*-regulating properties of the circulation, independent of external control mechanisms

2. to explain the need for external control mechanisms

3. to serve as a foundation on which we can construct a simple model of the control of circulation.

Our model is defined by the following equations (see Figure 5.6): First, we have the equations of the right and left hearts:

$$Q_r = K_r P_{sv} \qquad (5.5.1)$$

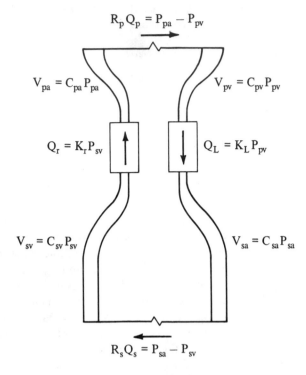

$$R_p Q_p = P_{pa} - P_{pv}$$

$$V_{pa} = C_{pa} P_{pa}$$

$$V_{pv} = C_{pv} P_{pv}$$

$$Q_r = K_r P_{sv}$$

$$Q_L = K_L P_{pv}$$

$$V_{sv} = C_{sv} P_{sv}$$

$$V_{sa} = C_{sa} P_{sa}$$

$$R_s Q_s = P_{sa} - P_{sv}$$

FIGURE 5.6.

$$Q_L = K_L P_{pv}. \tag{5.5.2}$$

Second, we make the assumption that the systemic and pulmonary arteries and veins are compliance vessels. For simplicity, we use (5.3.2) instead of (5.3.3). That is, we neglect V_d in these vessels. This gives the equations

$$V_{sa} = C_{sa} P_{sa} \tag{5.5.3}$$

$$V_{sv} = C_{sv} P_{sv} \tag{5.5.4}$$

$$V_{pa} = C_{pa} P_{pa} \tag{5.5.5}$$

$$V_{pv} = C_{pv} P_{pv}. \tag{5.5.6}$$

Third, we assume that the systemic and pulmonary tissues act like resistance vessels so that

$$Q_s = (1/R_s)(P_{sa} - P_{sv}) \tag{5.5.7}$$

$$Q_p = (1/R_p)(P_{pa} - P_{pv}). \tag{5.5.8}$$

At this point, we have an equation for each element of the circulation. Each equation contains a *parameter* that characterizes that element. These parameters are the pump coefficients K_r, K_L, the resistances R_s, R_p, and the compliances C_{sa}, C_{sv}, C_{pa}, and C_{pv}. Suppose we are given the values of these parameters. Can we use equations (5.5.1) through (5.5.8) to determine the flows, pressures and volumes of the model circulation? The answer to this question is negative; we do not yet have enough equations to determine the 12 unknowns

$$Q_r, Q_L, Q_s, Q_p; P_{sa}, P_{sv}, P_{pa}, P_{pv}; V_{sa}, V_{sv}, V_{pa}, V_{pv}.$$

The missing equations refer not to any particular element but to the circulation as a whole and to the way that its elements are connected. (Try to discover the missing equations for yourself before reading further.)

First, it is reasonable to assume that the total blood volume V_o is given. This gives the equation

$$V_{sa} + V_{sv} + V_{pa} + V_{pv} = V_o \tag{5.5.9}$$

in which V_o is an additional parameter.

Next, we assume that the circulation is in a *steady state*, so that the flow into each of the compliance vessels must equal the flow out (why?). It follows that $Q_r = Q_L = Q_s = Q_p$, so we can drop the subscripts and just refer to all of the flows as Q, the cardiac output.

With these additional assumptions, we have nine equations for nine unknowns $Q, P_{sa}, P_{sv}, P_{pa}, P_{pv}, V_{sa}, V_{sv}, V_{pa}, V_{pv}$. The model is complete.

Our next task is to solve the equations of the model. That is, we want to express each of the unknowns in terms of the parameters. (Try this for yourself before reading further.) An efficient plan of attack is as follows: First, express all of the pressures in terms of the flow Q. Then use the compliance equations to get the volumes in terms of Q. Finally, substitute in the equation for the total blood volume and solve for Q. With Q known (in terms of parameters only) we can go back and express the pressures and then the volumes in terms of parameters.

Here are the details. From the pump equations, we get the venous pressures in terms of Q:

$$P_{sv} = Q/Kr \tag{5.5.10}$$

$$P_{pv} = Q/K_L. \tag{5.5.11}$$

Substituting this result in the resistance equations, we get the arterial pressures in terms of Q:

$$P_{sa} = (Q/Kr) + R_s Q \tag{5.5.12}$$

$$P_{pa} = (Q/K_L) + R_p Q. \tag{5.5.13}$$

Substituting all four pressures into the compliance equations, we find

$$V_{sv} = (C_{sv}/K_r)Q \tag{5.5.14}$$

$$V_{pv} = (C_{pv}/K_L)Q \tag{5.5.15}$$

$$V_{sa} = [(C_{sa}/K_r) + C_{sa}R_s]Q \tag{5.5.16}$$

$$V_{pa} = [(C_{pa}/K_L) + C_{pa}R_p)]Q. \tag{5.5.17}$$

To save writing, we introduce the following combinations of parameters

$$T_{sv} = C_{sv}/K_r \tag{5.5.18}$$

$$T_{pv} = C_{pv}/K_L \tag{5.5.19}$$

$$T_{sa} = (C_{sa}/K_r) + C_{sa}R_s \tag{5.5.20}$$

$$T_{pa} = (C_{pa}/K_L) + C_{pa}R_p. \tag{5.5.21}$$

Then (5.5.14) through (5.5.17) can be summarized by the equations

$$V_i = T_i Q, \quad i = sv, pv, sa, pa. \tag{5.5.22}$$

We are now ready to substitute these expressions in the equations for the total blood volume and solve for Q. We get

$$(T_{sa} + T_{sv} + T_{pa} + T_{pv})Q = V_o \tag{5.5.23}$$

so

$$Q = V_o/(T_{sa} + T_{sv} + T_{pa} + T_{pv}). \tag{5.5.24}$$

The solution is completed using the equations $V_i = T_i Q$ and $P_i = V_i/C_i$. We get

$$V_i = T_i V_o/(T_{sa} + T_{sv} + T_{pa} + T_{pv}) \tag{5.5.25}$$

$$P_i = (1/C_i)(T_i V_o)/(T_{sa} + T_{sv} + T_{pa} + T_{pv}) \tag{5.5.26}$$

TABLE 5.2. Normal Resting Parameters of the Model Circulation

	Systemic	Pulmonary
R:	$R_s = 17.5$	$R_p = 1.79$ mm Hg/(liter/min)
C:	$C_{sa} = 0.01$	$C_{pa} = 0.00667$ liters/mm Hg
	$C_{sv} = 1.75$	$C_{pv} = 0.08$ liters/mm Hg

	Right	Left
K:	$K_r = 2.8$	$K_L = 1.12$ (liters/min)/mm Hg

V:	$V_o = 5.0$ liters

where $i = sa, sv, pa$, and pv. Thus, we have a formula for each unknown in terms of parameters only.

The quantitative use of these formulae depends on having numerical values for the parameters. In particular, we need *normal resting values* for the parameters so that we can use the model to predict the effects of parameter changes away from the normal resting state of the circulation. It is easy to determine the parameters from data such as are given in Table 5.1 and Section 5.2 because each equation of our model (5.5.1–5.5.9) contains exactly one of the parameters, so it can be written as a formula for that parameter in terms of the observed pressures, volumes, and flows. The results of this procedure are summarized in Table 5.2.

The procedure that we have just used for *identification* of parameters is based on the assumption that the model is correct. If we improve the model, then the best choice of parameters may change. An example of this is studied in Exercises 5.7 and 5.17.

5.6 Balancing the Two Sides of the Heart and the Two Circulations

The reader has probably noticed that most of the equations of the previous section came in pairs. The reason for this is the symmetry of form between the right and left heart and the systemic and pulmonary circulations. In fact, we can obtain one member of a pair from the other by making the subscript interchanges $s \leftrightarrow p$ and $r \leftrightarrow L$ (try it and see!). In the few equations that stand alone (because they refer to the circulation as a whole) these interchanges give us back the same equation as before.

If the corresponding parameters were quantitatively equal (that is, if we had $K_r = K_L, R_s = R_p$, etc.), then the two circulations would be quantitatively symmetrical with $P_{sa} = P_{pa}$, and so on. A glance at Tables 5.1 and 5.2 shows that this is far from being the case.

This raises the question of how the two sides of the heart and the two circulations are coordinated. What keeps the outputs of the right and left hearts equal? What mechanisms control the partition of blood volume between the systemic and pulmonary circulations? These are vital (and closely related) questions. If the left output exceeded the right output by only 10 % for 1 minute, this would be enough to empty the vessels of the pulmonary circulation.

In our steady state model of the circulation, the right and left cardiac outputs are equal by definition. In a time-dependent version of the model, we could see how this equality of output is maintained. Suppose, for example, that K_r is suddenly reduced. Temporarily, Q_r will be less than Q_L, so there will be a net transfer of blood volume away from the pulmonary circulation and into the systemic circulation. This will raise the systemic venous pressure and lower the pulmonary venous pressure. The effect of these pressure changes will be to drive the cardiac outputs back toward equality. A net rate of transfer of volume will persist until equality of output of the two sides has been restored. Then a new equilibrium is established with a different partition of the blood volume than before.

In the steady state model, we compute only the end result of this process. Using (5.5.25) and (5.5.18) through (5.5.21), we see that

$$V_p/V_s \;=\; (V_{pa} + V_{pv})/(V_{sa} + V_{sv})$$

$$=\; (T_{pa} + T_{pv})/(T_{sa} + T_{sv})$$

$$=\; ((C_{pa} + C_{pv})/K_L + C_{pa}R_p)/((C_{sa} + C_{sv})/Kr + C_{sa}R_s)$$
$$(5.6.1)$$

where V_p is the total pulmonary volume and V_s is the total systemic volume. Thus, the partition of the blood volume between the two circulations is determined by the parameters, and a change in parameters that temporarily produces a disparity in output between the two sides of the heart eventually results in a volume shift that compensates for the parameter change and restores the equality of output.

The key to the success of this intrinsic control mechanism is the dependence of *cardiac output* on *venous pressure*. Suppose instead that the cardiac outputs of the two sides of the heart were given and equal. In that case Q would be a parameter and we would have to drop Equations (5.5.1) and (5.5.2). We would have lost two equations but only one unknown, so we would be free to specify one more relationship. In fact, we could then assume that the pulmonary and systemic volumes (V_p, V_s) were separately given. This would lead to the equations

$$V_{sa} + V_{sv} = V_s \qquad\qquad (5.6.2)$$

$$V_{pa} + V_{pv} = V_p \qquad\qquad (5.6.3)$$

which would replace (5.5.9), increasing the number of equations by one. Thus, we would have eight equations (5.5.3) through (5.5.8) and (5.6.2) and (5.6.3) for the eight unknowns (V_i, P_i) with Q as a new parameter. With these assumptions the pulmonary and systemic volumes would be arbitrary; there would be no mechanism available to hold them in a reasonable relationship to each other. These considerations show the importance of the dependence of cardiac output on venous pressure, not only for maintaining a balance between the two sides of the heart, but also for establishing a controlled partition of the blood volume between the pulmonary and systemic circulations.

5.7   Cardiac Output and Arterial Blood Pressure: The Need or External Circulatory Control Mechanisms

The arterioles in an exercising muscle dilate and the systemic resistance R_s falls. The cardiac output rises and the systemic arterial pressure is maintained. The increase in cardiac output comes primarily from an increase in heart rate while stroke volume remains fairly constant.

In this section, we will study the consequences of a change in R_s in our model of the *uncontrolled* circulation. We will find a predicted response that is very different from the observed response described above. In the uncontrolled circulation a decrease in R_s results in only a modest increase in cardiac output. The most noticeable effect is a substantial fall in systemic arterial pressure. This shows the need for the external circulatory control mechanisms that are outlined in the next section.

We begin with an obvious but important remark. The effects of a change in R_s cannot be predicted solely from the equation of the systemic resistance, even though that is the only equation where R_s appears. If we neglect P_{sv} in Equation (5.5.7) (an excellent approximation because P_{sv} is about 2 mm Hg whereas P_{sa} is about 100 mm Hg), we get $P_{sa} = Q \, R_s$. From this we might conclude that P_{sa} is proportional to R_s with Q constant or that Q is inversely proportional to R_s with P_{sa} constant. Neither conclusion is correct since both P_{sa} and Q vary when R_s changes. The actual effects on P_{sa} and Q cannot be predicted without taking all of the other equations into account. That is the essence of a system of *simultaneous* equations.

In fact, we have already taken these equations into account when we solved for the unknowns in terms of the parameters. The formulae that we need are

$$Q = V_o/(T_{sa} + T_{sv} + T_{pa} + T_{pv}) \tag{5.7.1}$$

and

$$P_{sa} = (V_o/C_{sa})(T_{sa}/(T_{sa} + T_{sv} + T_{pa} + T_{pv})) \tag{5.7.2}$$

where T_{sa}, etc., are given by (5.5.18) through (5.5.21).

Using these formulae and the parameter values given in Table 5.2, we can find the effects on Q and P_{sa} of reducing R_s to 50% of its normal value (while

TABLE 5.3. Effect of Changing Systemic Resistance on Cardiac Output and Systemic Arterial Pressure in the Uncontrolled Circulation

	Normal	$R_s = R_s^{normal}/2$	Change	% Change
Q	5.6	6.2	+0.6 liters/min	+11%
P_{sa}	100.0	57	-43.0 mm Hg	-43%

leaving the other parameters unchanged). The results are summarized in Table 5.3.

Note that the increase in cardiac output was only about 10% whereas the drop in arterial pressure was about 40%. This mechanism of adjusting the cardiac output is definitely inadequate to sustain reasonable levels of exercise, where cardiac output must be doubled or even tripled and where blood supply to nonmuscular tissue must be maintained.

The results that we have just derived can be summarized using the concept of sensitivity. If Y depends on X, and X changes, then the sensitivity of Y to X is defined to be

$$
\begin{aligned}
\sigma_{YX} &= \Delta \log(Y)/\Delta \log(X) = (\log(Y') - \log(Y))/(\log(X') - \log(X)) \\
&= \log(Y'/Y)/\log(X'/X)
\end{aligned}
$$

$$(5.7.3)$$

where $X' = X + \Delta X$ and Y' is the value that Y takes on when X is changed to X'. Note that the sensitivity is not influenced by a change of units in X or Y. It also makes no difference what base is used for the logarithms in these formulae. When the changes in X and Y are small, we have approximately

$$\sigma_{YX} = (dY/Y)/(dX/X) \tag{5.7.4}$$

which shows that the sensitivity is roughly the ratio of relative (or %) changes. If $Y = a X^n$, then $\log Y = n \log X$ and $\sigma_{YX} = n$. In particular, if Y is proportional to X, then $\sigma_{YX} = 1$. If Y is inversely proportional to X, then $\sigma_{YX} = -1$.

From the numbers in Table 5.3, we conclude that $\sigma_{QR_s} = -0.15$ while $\sigma_{P_{sa}R_s} = +0.81$. It is not a coincidence that

$$-(\sigma_{QR_s}) + \sigma_{P_{sa}R_s} \cong 1 \tag{5.7.5}$$

This follows from the fact that $P_{sa} \cong QR_s$ as the reader can show by taking logarithms and applying the definition of sensitivity. Because of (5.7.5), we cannot increase the magnitude of the sensitivity of cardiac output to systemic resistance without *decreasing* the sensitivity of systemic arterial pressure to systemic resistance. Any mechanism that accomplishes one will automatically accomplish the other.

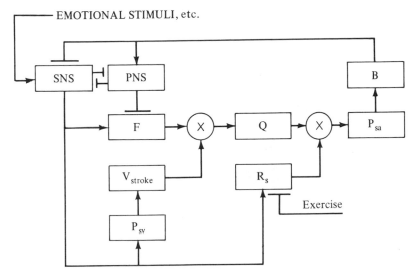

FIGURE 5.7.

5.8   Neural Control: The Baroreceptor Loop

From the results of the previous section, it appears that it would be a good idea to hold P_{sa} constant. In that case, we should have $\sigma_{P_{sa}R_s} = 0$ and $\sigma_{QR_s} = -1$, which would be a tremendous improvement from the standpoint of the circulatory response to exercise. The improvement would be twofold. First, $\sigma_{QR_s} = -1$ would mean that the cardiac output would double every time the systemic resistance were halved. Second, $\sigma_{QR_s} = 0$ would mean that the systemic arterial pressure (and hence the blood flow to the non-exercising tissues and organs) would be maintained.

In the body, P_{sa} is controlled by a feedback mechanism called the baroreceptor loop (see Figure 5.7, in which an arrow indicates a positive or excitatory influence and a bar indicates a negative or inhibitory influence). The elements of the baroreceptor loop are as follows:

1. The *baroreceptors* (B) are stretch receptors located in the carotid arteries and in the arch of the aorta. The baroreceptors transmit nerve impulses to the brain stem at a rate that increases with increasing arterial pressure (see Chapter 10).

2. The *parasympathetic nervous system* (PNS) is excited by activity of the baroreceptors. Its effect is to slow the heart rate (F).

3. The *sympathetic nervous system* (SNS) is inhibited by activity of the baroreceptors. It has several effects on the circulation, including:

a. increased heart rate

b. increased venous pressure, and so increased stroke volume

c. increased systemic resistance.

The loop is closed through the mechanics of the circulation which imply that $Q = FV_{stroke}$ and that $P_{sa} = Q\,R_s$.

Tracing any closed loop from P_{sa} back to P_{sa} in Figure 5.7, we find an odd number of inhibitory influences. This means that any changes in P_{sa} lead to *compensatory* changes through the baroreceptor loop.

We will not present a detailed model of the baroreceptor loop here (see Chapter 10 however). Instead, we model its overall function by assuming that the baroreceptor loop adjusts the heart rate F until the systemic arterial pressure achieves a target value P^*. Note that this model ignores the effects of the sympathetic nervous system on venous pressure and on systemic resistance. These effects are less important than the effect on heart rate in the normal operation of the circulation.

Thus, we have a new unknown, F, that was previously a parameter and a new parameter, $P_{sa} = P^*$, that was previously an unknown. Also, because F is no longer a parameter, we have to rewrite (5.5.1) and (5.5.2) in the form

$$Q_r = F\,C_r\,P_{sv} \tag{5.8.1}$$

$$Q_L = F\,C_L\,P_{pv} \tag{5.8.2}$$

where C_r and C_L are the *diastolic compliance* of the right and left hearts (see Section 5.4), so that C_rP_{sv} is the right stroke volume and C_LP_{pv} is the left stroke volume.

This gives us a model of the controlled circulation in which the equations are (5.8.1) and (5.8.2) together with (5.5.3) through (5.5.9) and the steady state relation $Q_r = Q_p = Q_s = Q_L$. The unknowns are the same as before except that now F replaces P_{sa}.

Instead of solving these equations directly, we make some approximations. First, we neglect P_{sv} compared to P_{sa} in the equation of the systemic resistance. This represents a 2% error, and it gives us the equation

$$Q\,R_s = P^*. \tag{5.8.3}$$

Next, we neglect the pulmonary volumes in comparison with the systemic volumes in the equation of the total blood volume. This represents a 10% error, and it gives us

$$V_{sa} + V_{sv} = V_o \tag{5.8.4}$$

which can be rewritten

$$C_{sa}P^* + C_{sv}P_{sv} = V_o. \tag{5.8.5}$$

We can now determine Q directly from (5.8.3) and P_{sv} directly from (5.8.5):

$$Q = P^*/R_s \tag{5.8.6}$$

$$P_{sv} = (V_o - C_{sa}P^*)/C_{sv}.$$ (5.8.7)

Substituting these results in the equation of the right heart (5.8.1), we can solve for the heart rate

$$F = P^*C_{sv}/(R_sC_r(V_o - C_{sa}P^*)).$$ (5.8.8)

These results summarize the performance of the controlled circulation. We have achieved what we set out to do: Since $P_{sa} = P^*$, which is constant, $\sigma_{P_{sa}R_s} = 0$. Again, since P^* is constant, $\sigma_{QR_s} = -1$.

Thus, our model of the controlled circulation responds to changes in R_s with (inversely) proportional changes in cardiac output while the arterial pressure is maintained. In the model as in life, the mechanism responsible for the increased cardiac output is an increase in heart rate, since the venous pressure and stroke volume ($V_{stroke} = C_rP_{sv}$) are independent of R_s in the model.

In the uncontrolled circulation the cardiac output depends on all of the parameters of the model; in the controlled circulation it only depends on Γ^* and R_s. This isolation of cardiac output from extraneous influences is just as important as the heightened sensitivity to R_s. We give one example. In the uncontrolled circulation, we had $\sigma_{QV_o} = 1$, which means that the cardiac output is proportional to the blood volume (see Equation 5.5.24). In the controlled circulation, $\sigma_{QV_o} = 0$, which means that the cardiac output is protected against blood loss, for example. From (5.8.8), we see that the mechanism of adaptation to blood loss is an increase in heart rate that compensates for the decrease in stroke volume. We also see that the model breaks down when $V_o = C_{sa}P^*$, which corresponds to complete depletion of the systemic venous blood.

We have shown that the response of the controlled circulation to stress is very different from that of the uncontrolled circulation. It is remarkable that such dramatic changes in behavior emerge when the only change in the mathematical model is to make one parameter into an unknown and one unknown into a parameter.

5.9 Autoregulation

Up to this point, we have treated the systemic resistance as a parameter. In this section, we will consider the local control of systemic resistance. Central control of systemic resistance was mentioned, but not modeled, in the previous section (see also Chapter 10).

There are two phenomena that come under the term autoregulation:

1. When the pressure–flow relation of a tissue is measured, it often turns out that there is a range of pressures in which the flow is relatively insensitive to the pressure difference.

2. At constant pressure difference, the flow through many tissues depends on the rate of O_2 consumption of the tissue.

In the normal function of the circulation, the second phenomenon is more important than the first, since the pressure difference is relatively constant, as we have just seen in the previous section. In pathological conditions, the first phenomenon may be important for regulating blood flow in the face of fluctuating pressures.

In this section we outline a simple model that accounts for both phenomena through a single mechanism. The model that we shall describe is a simplified version of a model proposed by Huntsman, Attinger, and Noordergraaf.

The key hypothesis is that the resistance of a tissue is regulated by the venous O_2 concentration of the tissue. In general, *concentration* means the amount per unit volume, and its units depend on how the amount is measured. In the case of a gas, it is convenient to measure the amount of gas in terms of the volume that the gas would occupy under some specified conditions of temperature and pressure. In physiology, the most natural conditions are atmospheric pressure and body temperature. When this is done, the concentration becomes dimensionless (volume/volume.)

For example, the concentration of O_2 in blood, denoted by $[O_2]$, is the number of liters of O_2 that are carried in one liter of blood. Oxygen is carried in blood bound to hemoglobin, and when all of the O_2-carrying sites in the hemoglobin molecules are occupied, the concentration of O_2 in blood is $\frac{1}{5}$. Coincidentally, this is the same as the concentration of O_2 in the atmosphere itself. Under normal conditions, the hemoglobin becomes saturated as it passes through the lungs so that the arterial concentration $[O_2]_a = \frac{1}{5}$. The O_2 concentration of arterial blood is, of course, constant for all of the tissues of the body, but it may vary under conditions of high altitude or anemia. In the former case, the hemoglobin may fail to be saturated in the lung. In the latter case, the concentration of hemoglobin in blood is lower than normal. In both cases, $[O_2]_a$ is reduced, but this reduction is felt by all tissues of the body.

The venous O_2 concentration, $[O_2]_v$, is different in the different tissues of the body. Let M (metabolic rate) stand for the rate of O_2 consumption of a tissue. M has units of liters/minute. Also, let Q be the blood flow to the tissue in question. The rate at which O_2 is delivered to the tissue in the arterial blood is $Q[O_2]_a$, the units of which are (liters of blood/minute) × (liters of O_2/liter of blood). Similarly, the rate at which O_2 leaves the tissue in its venous blood is $Q[O_2]_v$. If the tissue is in a steady state, the difference must be accounted for by the metabolic rate of the tissue. This gives the equation

$$Q[O_2]_a - Q[O_2]_v = M \qquad (5.9.1)$$

which is called the *Fick Principle*. Thus,

$$[O_2]_v = [O_2]_a - M/Q. \qquad (5.9.2)$$

This formula shows that $[O_2]_v$ may serve as an index of the adequacy of the blood supply in relation to the metabolic rate of the tissues. When the blood supply is just barely sufficient to sustain the metabolic rate

$$Q = Q^* = M/[O_2]_a \quad \text{(this defines } Q^*\text{)} \tag{5.9.3}$$

and we get $[O_2]_v = 0$. As Q is raised above Q^*, $[O_2]_v$ rises and finally $[O_{O2}]_v \to [O_2]_a$ as $Q \to \infty$. This shows why it might be reasonable to use $[O_2]_v$ to regulate the resistance of a tissue to blood flow.

A problem with this hypothesis is that resistance is regulated on the arterial side of the tissue, not on the venous side. The venous O_2 concentration is determined by the *tissue* O_2 concentration, however, and the arterioles run through the tissue and may therefore be influenced by the tissue O_2 concentration.

Suppose, for example, that

$$R = R_o[O_2]_v \tag{5.9.4}$$

where

$$R = P/Q \tag{5.9.5}$$

is the resistance of the tissue to blood flow, P is the arteriovenous pressure difference ($P = P_{sa} - P_{sv}$), and R_o is the constant of proportionality that relates the resistance of the tissue to the venous O_2 concentration.

Equation (5.9.4) simply asserts that tissue resistance to blood flow is proportional to venous O_2 concentration. This is the simplest of a class of models in which tissue resistance is regulated by venous O_2 concentration.

To study the consequences of this simple hypothesis, we substitute (5.9.2) and (5.9.5) into (5.9.4) to obtain the pressure–flow relation of a tissue in which resistance is regulated in this way. The result is

$$Q = M/[O_2]_a + P/(R_o[O_2]_a) \tag{5.9.6}$$

$$= Q^* + P/(R_o[O_2]_a) \tag{5.9.7}$$

where $Q^* = M/[O_2]_a$. This result is plotted in Figure 5.8. The behavior of the model tissue is summarized by the following statements, which the reader should be able to verify:

1. The sensitivity of flow to pressure (σ_{QP}) is less when $R = R_o[O_2]_v$ than when $R = $ constant.

2. The tissue always receives at least the minimum flow Q^* required to sustain its metabolic rate. (Think about how this works. When $P \to 0$, why doesn't $Q \to 0$ in the model? What happens to R and $[O_2]_v$?)

3. At constant P, if M changes then $\Delta Q = \Delta Q^* = \Delta M/[O_2]_a$. This means that the change in blood flow is just what is needed to support the extra O_2 consumption.

4. At constant P, if M increases, then R automatically decreases. (Plot R as a function of M with P, $[O_2]_a$ and R_o constant.)

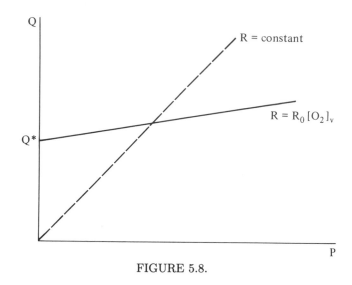

FIGURE 5.8.

5. If $[O_2]_a$ changes (with P and R_o constant) then Q automatically adjusts in such a way that $Q[O_2]_a = $ constant. Therefore, the rate of O_2 supply to all of the tissues is the same as it was before the change in $[O_2]_a$.

In summary, the simple device of setting $R = R_o[O_2]_v$ (instead of $R = $ constant) makes the blood supply to a tissue less sensitive to pressure changes and more responsive to the needs of the tissue.

5.10   Changes in the Circulation Occurring at Birth

The circulation forms a simple loop after birth. Before birth, however, the configuration of the circulation is complicated by additional connections. One of these is a vessel called the *ductus arteriosus*, which connects the pulmonary and systemic arteries near the heart. Another is an opening in the wall that separates the right and left atria. This opening, called the *foramen ovale*, is guarded by a flap of tissue that acts as a valve to ensure that blood flow through the foramen always goes from right to left.

The function of these extra connections is to shunt blood away from the lungs, which are collapsed before birth and which therefore present high resistance to blood flow.

In this section, we will present a simple model of the *fetal circulation* (the circulation before birth), and we will use this model to explain the sequence of changes (initiated by the first breath) that close the shunts and establish the single-loop configuration of the circulation that persists into adult life.

The model is shown in Figure 5.9. The shunt flows are the ductus flow Q_d and the foramen flow Q_f. If these are both zero, then the model takes on the configuration of a simple loop in which blood flows through the right heart;

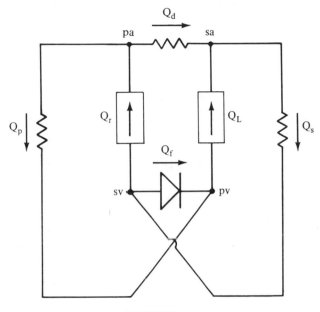

FIGURE 5.9.

the pulmonary arteries, tissues, and veins; the left heart; and the systemic arteries, tissues, and veins.

Note that the flow through the ductus arteriosus is not always in the direction indicated by the arrow in Figure 5.9. The arrow points in the direction of the flow that we have elected to call positive, which is also the normal direction of flow during fetal life. After birth but before the closure of the ductus arteriosus, however, the flow through the ductus is in the opposite direction. The reasons for this sudden reversal at birth will be explained below. The two situations are easily accommodated by a single system of equations if we consider the reverse flow through the ductus as being negative. Thus, $Q_d > 0$ means that the flow is in the direction defined by the arrow in Figure 5.9, whereas $Q_d < 0$ means that flow is in the opposite direction.

The equations we use are those of the uncontrolled circulation:

$$Q_r = K_r P_{sv} \tag{5.10.1}$$

$$Q_L = K_L P_{pv} \tag{5.10.2}$$

$$Q_p = (P_{pa} - P_{pv})/R_p \tag{5.10.3}$$

$$Q_s = (P_{sa} - P_{sv})/R_s \tag{5.10.4}$$

which must be supplemented by the equations for the ductus and the foramen. The ductus is modeled as being a simple resistance

$$Q_d = (P_{pa} - P_{sa})/R_d. \tag{5.10.5}$$

The foramen is modeled as an ideal valve. This means that the valve may be *open*, in which case

$$Q_f \geq 0 \quad \text{and} \quad P_{sv} = P_{pv} \tag{5.10.6}$$

or *closed*, in which case

$$Q_f = 0 \quad \text{and} P_{sv} \leq P_{pv}. \tag{5.10.7}$$

Unfortunately, the natural terminology for a fluid valve is precisely the opposite of the natural terminology for an electrical switch, where "closed" means conducting and "open" means nonconducting. We shall use the natural fluid terminology here, with apologies for the confusion that this may cause to the reader who is accustomed to the electrical terminology.

How do we decide whether the foramen is open or closed? The answer is to try either alternative and see whether or not it is self-consistent. For example, we could start by assuming the foramen is open and use the equation $P_{sv} = P_{pv}$. This will give enough equations to determine Q_f and we can check whether or not $Q_f \geq 0$. If not, our original guess was incorrect. (The reader may want to worry about what to do if both assumptions or neither turn out to be self-consistent. Such concern is unnecessary because of the following theorem, which the reader may enjoy trying to prove: For any set of parameter values, at least one of the conditions (5.10.6) or (5.10.7) is self-consistent, and if both are self-consistent the parameters must be such that $P_{sv} = P_{pv}$ and $Q_f = 0$. In the latter case, it makes no difference whether we say that the foramen is open or closed.)

We now have equations for each element of the model, but we need the steady state relationships among the different flows. In the nonfetal circulation, these relationships were very simple ($Q_r = Q_L = Q_p = Q_s$), and there was really only one independent flow, the cardiac output. Here, the situation is much more complicated.

At each junction in Figure 5.9, we have the relationship that the total flow *in* equals the total flow *out*. This gives the following four equations:

$$pa : Q_r = Q_p + Q_d \tag{5.10.8}$$

$$sa : Q_d + Q_L = Q_s \tag{5.10.9}$$

$$sv : Q_s = Q_r + Q_f \tag{5.10.10}$$

$$pv : Q_p + Q_f = Q_L. \tag{5.10.11}$$

Note that each of the six flows appears exactly once on the left-hand side and exactly once on the right-hand side of Equations (5.10.8) through (5.10.11). (Why?) Thus, the sum of these four equations gives an identity

$$Q_r + Q_d + Q_L + Q_s + Q_p + Q_f = Q_r + Q_d + Q_L + Q_s + Q_p + Q_f.$$

It follows that any one of these equations can be derived from the other three. (Try it and see.) In short, we have three independent relations among six flows in the model, so we can express all of the flows in terms of any three of them. If we (arbitrarily) choose Q_r, Q_d, Q_L as these three flows, then we have as a consequence of (5.10.8) through (5.10.11) that

$$Q_s = Q_L + Q_d \tag{5.10.12}$$

$$Q_p = Q_r - Q_d \tag{5.10.13}$$

$$Q_f = Q_L - Q_r + Q_d. \tag{5.10.14}$$

The last equation shows the importance of having both an arterial and an atrial (venous) shunt. If we want $Q_r = Q_L$, then we must have $Q_f = Q_d$. Conversely, if Q_d or Q_f is zero, then an imbalance between the two sides of the heart will be required to shunt blood away from the lungs. Presumably, it is important to maintain at least a rough equality of output between the two sides of the heart during fetal life in order that the heart should develop properly and be prepared for the postnatal situation in which the configuration of the circulation is a single closed loop and in which both sides of the heart must therefore pump the same amount of blood per unit time. As we have just shown, the need to shunt blood away from the high-resistance fetal lungs can only be reconciled with the need to balance the outputs of the two sides of the heart if *two* shunts are provided, one on the venous side (the foramen ovale) and one on the arterial side (the ductus arteriosus).

We are now ready to solve the equations of the fetal circulation. First, we remark that the fetal circulation is characterized by a high pulmonary resistance (because the lungs are collapsed) and a low systemic resistance (because of blood flow to the placenta through the umbilical cord). The result is that $R_p > R_s$, a relationship that reverses after birth. A second remark is that the two sides of the heart are more nearly equal in their compliance properties before birth than afterwards. We model this by setting

$$K_r = K_L = K \quad \text{(this defines } K\text{)}.$$

Third, the ductus is wide open before birth, and we assume that $R_d = 0$. This gives the equation

$$P_{sa} = P_{pa} = P_a \quad \text{(this defines } P_a\text{)}. \tag{5.10.16}$$

Finally, we make the provisional assumption that the foramen ovale is open before birth. This gives the equation

$$P_{sv} = P_{pv} = P_v \quad \text{(this defines } P_v\text{)}. \tag{5.10.17}$$

Later, we will have to solve for Q_f and check that $Q_f \geq 0$.

The analysis of the model is now simple. Since there is a common venous pressure and the two sides of the heart are the same ($K_r = K_L$), we have

$$K P_v = Q_r = Q_L = Q \quad \text{(this defines } Q\text{)}. \tag{5.10.18}$$

Since there is also a common arterial pressure, we have

$$R_s Q_s = R_p Q_p = P_a - P_v. \tag{5.10.19}$$

Thus, the ratio of the pulmonary to the systemic flow is controlled (inversely) by the ratio of resistances

$$Q_p/Q_s = R_s/R_p. \tag{5.10.20}$$

Using (5.10.12) through (5.10.14), we get

$$(Q - Q_d)/(Q + Q_d) = R_s/R_p \tag{5.10.21}$$

which can be solved for Q_d/Q:

$$Q_d/Q = (R_p - R_s)/(R_p + R_s) \tag{5.10.22}$$

The foramen flow is determined by (5.10.14) which reduces to $Q_f = Q_d$ since $Q_r = Q_L$. Thus, we also have

$$Q_f/Q = (R_p - R_s)/(R_p + R_s). \tag{5.10.23}$$

Finally, from equations (5.10.12) and (5.10.13), we see that

$$Q_s/Q = 1 + Q_d/Q = 1 + (R_p - R_s)/(R_p + R_s) = 2R_p/(R_p + R_s) \tag{5.10.24}$$

$$Q_p/Q = 1 - Q_d/Q = 1 - (R_p - R_s)/(R_p + R_s) = 2R_s/(R_p + R_s). \tag{5.10.25}$$

We have now determined all of the ratios of flows in the model in terms of the parameters R_p and R_s. Note that $Q_f > 0$ as long as $R_p > R_s$, so we have found a self-consistent solution with the foramen ovale *open*.

Perhaps the best way to appreciate the effectiveness of the model in shunting blood flow away from the high resistance lungs is to consider the extreme case $R_p = \infty$. None of our formulae yield infinite values in this case. We simply get the limiting solution $Q_f = Q_d = Q, Q_s = 2Q$, and $Q_p = 0$.

At birth, the lungs expand with the first breath, and R_p falls suddenly. The umbilical cord constricts (either naturally or because it is clamped) and R_s rises suddenly. The net effect is that $R_p < R_s$. This makes $Q_f < 0$ in (5.10.23). This means that the solution found above is no longer self-consistent. Therefore, the flap of tissue guarding the foramen ovale suddenly slams shut.

A closed foramen, self-consistent solution is found in the Exercises at the end of the Chapter. This describes the circulation after birth when $R_p < R_s$. One property of this solution is $Q_d < 0$, which means that the flow in the ductus has reversed compared to the fetal case. After birth the flow through the ductus is a *left-to-right shunt* and it carries fully oxygenated blood from the aorta back into the pulmonary arterial tree. The high O_2 content of this blood stimulates the closure of the ductus, completing the transition to a single-loop circulation.

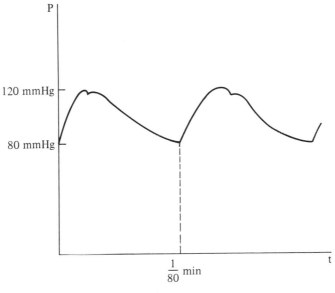

FIGURE 5.10.

5.11 Dynamics of the Arterial Pulse

In the foregoing sections, we have treated the circulation as though all of the pressures, flows and volumes are constant in time. This is not correct. Actually, the heart ejects blood into the arteries in discrete bursts. During these contractions of the heart, the blood pressure rises rapidly, and it falls again between contractions as blood runs out of the arteries through the tissues. The result of this process is the *arterial pulse*, which can be felt wherever an artery is convenient to press (e.g., at the wrist) and which can be used to count the heart rate. The wave form of the arterial pulse is sketched in Figure 5.10.

When blood pressure is measured with an air cuff on the upper arm, the actual quantities determined by this measurement are the maximum (systolic) and minimum (diastolic) pressures achieved by the arterial pulse. A blood pressure of 120/80 means that the systolic arterial blood pressure is 120 mm Hg and the diastolic arterial blood pressure is 80 mm Hg. The difference between these values (in this case 40 mm Hg) is called the *pulse pressure*.

The names *systolic* and *diastolic* refer to the phases of the cardiac cycle (see Section 5.4). Under normal conditions, the systolic pressure in the systemic arteries is essentially the same as the systolic left ventricular pressure, since the aortic valve is open during systole. The diastolic pressure in the ventricle is much lower than that in the arteries. This is possible because the aortic valve is closed during diastole.

In this section, we shall describe the simplest model that can account for the qualitative form of the arterial pulse. This model will be used to show how

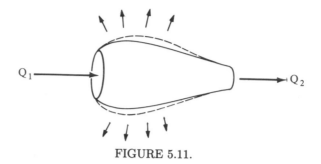

FIGURE 5.11.

the systolic and diastolic pressures depend on the parameters of the heart and circulation. It will also be used to justify the simpler steady flow models that were studied in the foregoing sections of this chapter.

We begin by considering a compliance vessel that is not in the steady state (see Figure 5.11). Thus, the inflow $Q_1(t)$ is not equal to the outflow $Q_2(t)$ at every instant. When they are not equal, the volume of the vessel changes. In fact, if $V(t)$ denotes the volume of the vessel at time t, we have

$$dV/dt = Q_1 - Q_2. \tag{5.11.1}$$

This says that the rate of change of the vessel's volume is the difference between the flow in and the flow out. When $V = $ constant, $Q_1 = Q_2$, which is the steady state relation that we have used up to now.

This differential equation describes how the volume changes, but it can be converted into one relating the pressure in the vessel to the flows in and out by using the equation of a compliance vessel: Either

$$V(t) = C\,P(t) \quad \text{or} \quad V(t) = C\,P(t) + V_d$$

(see Section 5.3). In either case, we have $dV/dt = C\,dP/dt$, so

$$C\,dP/dt = Q_1 - Q_2. \tag{5.11.2}$$

This is the equation that governs pressure changes in a compliance vessel in the case of unsteady flow.

Next, we use this equation to study the systemic arterial tree. Now, $P = P_{sa}$, the systemic arterial pressure; $C = C_{sa}$ the systemic arterial compliance, $Q_1 = Q_L$ the output of the left heart, and $Q_2 = Q_s$, the blood flow through the systemic tissues. For Q_s, we have the equation $Q_s = (P_{sa} - P_{sv})/R_s$, which we approximate by

$$Q_s = P_{sa}/R_s \tag{5.11.3}$$

since $P_{sv} \ll P_{sa}$. Thus, (5.11.2) becomes

$$C_{sa}dP_{sa}/dt = Q_L(t) - P_{sa}/R_s \tag{5.11.4}$$

During diastole, when the aortic valve is closed, $Q_L = 0$. In that case, the solution of (5.11.4) is

$$P_{sa}(t) = P_{sa}(0)\exp(-t/(R_sC_{sa})). \tag{5.11.5}$$

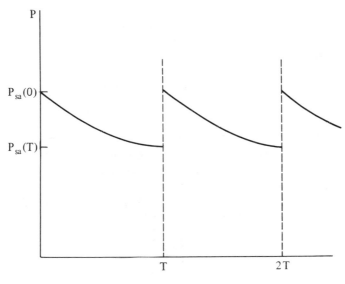

FIGURE 5.12.

The constant $P_{sa}(0)$ remains to be determined.

To find it, we consider ventricular systole. We make the simplifying assumption that the entire stroke volume ΔV_o is ejected from the heart instantaneously. Then we cannot use Equation (5.11.4) for systole. When ejection is idealized as being instantaneous, the flow $Q_L(t)$ is infinite for zero time during each systole, but in such a way that the integral of $Q_L(t)$ over each systole is the finite stroke volume ΔV_o. There is a mathematical device for dealing with this situation; it is called the *Dirac delta function*. If we were to write $Q_L(t)$ in terms of delta functions, we could retain the use of Equation (5.11.4) even in the case of instantaneous ejection. Here, however, we adopt a more elementary approach as follows. First, we find the change in pressure produced in the arteries by a sudden change in volume of magnitude ΔV_o: From the compliance equation $V = C\,P + V_d$, it is clear that

$$\Delta V_o = C_{sa}\Delta P_{sa}. \tag{5.11.6}$$

Now suppose that the heartbeat is a *periodic* phenomenon. That is, suppose that everything repeats exactly from one beat to the next. Let the duration of each heartbeat be T, so that the heart rate is $1/T$. Then the diastolic arterial pressure is $P_{sa}(T)$ and the systolic arterial pressure is $P_{sa}(0)$ (see Figure 5.12). Thus, the jump in pressure caused by cardiac ejection is given by the formula

$$\Delta P_{sa} = P_{sa}(0) - P_{sa}(T). \tag{5.11.7}$$

Now let $t = T$ in (5.11.5) and substitute (5.11.7) into (5.11.6) to obtain a pair of equations for $P_{sa}(0)$ and $P_{sa}(T)$. The result is

$$P_{sa}(T) = \Theta P_{sa}(0) \tag{5.11.8}$$

$$\Delta V_o/C_{sa} = P_{sa}(0) - P_{sa}(T) \tag{5.11.9}$$

where

$$\Theta = \exp(-T/(R_s C_{sa})) \tag{5.11.10}$$

Note that $0 < \Theta < 1$. Solving these equations gives

$$P_{sa}(0) = \Delta V_o/(C_{sa}(1 - \Theta)) \tag{5.11.11}$$

$$P_{sa}(T) = \Delta V_o\Theta/(C_{sa}(1 - \Theta)) \tag{5.11.12}$$

which are formulae for the systolic and diastolic pressures in terms of the stroke volume, the arterial compliance, the systemic resistance, and the heart rate. Subtracting these two equations, we recover (5.11.9), which is the formula for the pulse pressure.

What about the mean arterial pressure? A useful definition of the *mean* of a periodic function, say $f(t)$, is

$$< f >= \frac{1}{T} \int_0^T f(t)\, dt$$

where the period of f is T and where integration is over any period, e.g. over the interval $(0, T)$. With this notation, we define the mean arterial pressure to be

$$< P_{sa} >= \frac{1}{T} \int_0^T P_{sa}(t)\, dt. \tag{5.11.13}$$

(This is approximately the average of N samples of the function $P_{sa}(t)$ taken at equally spaced times that span the interval $[0, T]$. The approximation becomes exact as $N \to \infty$.) We leave it as an exercise to check that

$$< P_{sa} >= \Delta V_o R_s/T. \tag{5.11.14}$$

Since $\Delta V_o/T$ is the cardiac output, this equation can be interpreted as $< P_{sa} >= Q\, R_s$, which is the equation that holds in the steady state case (if we neglect P_{sv} as we are doing here). This explains how a steady state model still has significance for a pulsatile circulation: The quantities appearing in the steady state model are the time-averages of the corresponding pulsatile quantities.[1]

We have determined the form of the arterial pulse in the periodic case, where everything repeats exactly from one beat to the next. This is not quite correct even in the normal circulation where the heart rate and stroke volumes change

---

[1]This statement is only approximate. In a pulsatile version of the whole circulation model considered above, the pressures that determine the cardiac outputs would be the end-diastolic venous pressures, not the mean pressures, since it is the end-diastolic pressures that determine the volumes of the ventricular chambers just prior to ejection. More generally, any nonlinearity that might be introduced to make the model more realistic would further degrade the correspondence between the steady flow results and the mean values of the pulsatile results.

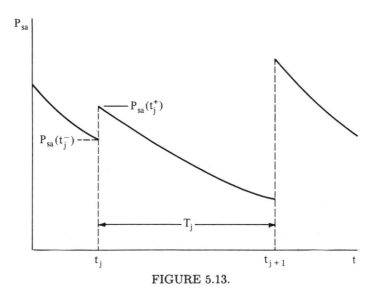

FIGURE 5.13.

slightly in response to the phases of breathing. The assumption of periodicity is even less appropriate for individuals with abnormal rhythms of the heart where successive heartbeats may be considerably different from each other, both in their durations and in their stroke volumes. As an extreme example of a nonperiodic arterial pulse, consider what happens if the heart has just been started following a period of cardiac arrest. The arterial pressure is initially very low and it has to build up toward its equilibrium values over the first few beats. The rest of this section studies these transient situations.

If the stroke volume and timing vary from beat to beat, we need notation to tell us what happens on each beat. Let $j = 1, 2, \ldots$, be an index counting beats of the heart. Let t_j be the time that the jth beat occurs, and let ΔV_j be the corresponding stroke volume. Since the pressure $P_{sa}(t)$ jumps at the times t_j (see Figure 5.13), we need notation to distinguish the arterial pressures just before and just after cardiac ejection. Let

$P_{sa}(t_j^-)$ = Arterial pressure just before ejection (diastolic)

$P_{sa}(t_j^+)$ = Arterial pressure just after ejection (systolic)

Between beats of the heart, we have, as before, the differential equation

$$C_{sa} dP_{sa}/dt = -P_{sa}/R_s$$

but now, it is more convenient to write the solutions in the form

$$P_{sa}(t) = P_{sa}(t_j^+) \exp(-(t - t_j)/(R_s C_{sa})) \tag{5.11.15}$$

$$\text{for } t_j < t < t_{j+1}.$$

Setting $t = t_{j+1}^-$ gives

$$P_{sa}(t_{j+1}^-) = P_{sa}(t_j^+)\Theta_j \tag{5.11.16}$$

where

$$\Theta_j = \exp(-T_j/(R_s C_{sa})) \qquad (5.11.17)$$

and

$$T_j = t_{j+1} - t_j. \qquad (5.11.18)$$

Equation (5.11.16) gives the diastolic pressure just before beat $j+1$ in terms of the systolic pressure just after beat j.

The equation for the jump in arterial pressure on beat j now takes the form

$$P_{sa}(t_j^+) = P_{sa}(t_j^-) + \Delta V_j/C_{sa}. \qquad (5.11.19)$$

Now suppose that we are given any sequence of times t_j and stroke volumes ΔV_j together with the constant parameters C_{sa} and R_s. If we are told the diastolic pressure just before the first beat, we can use (5.11.19) to find the systolic pressure just after that beat. Then we can use (5.11.16) to find the diastolic pressure just before the next beat. Repeating this process we can predict the entire sequence of diastolic and systolic pressures, however irregular it might be.

The equations that we have just developed for the nonperiodic situation should include the periodic arterial pulse as a special case. Suppose the heartbeat is regular so that $t_{j+1} - t_j = T$ and $\Delta V_j = \Delta V_o$ for all j. Then Θ_j reduces to Θ and equations (5.11.16) and (5.11.19) become

$$P_{sa}(t_{j+1}^-) = P_{sa}(t_j^+)\Theta \qquad (5.11.20)$$

$$P_{sa}(t_j^+) = Psa(t_j^-) + \Delta V_o/C_{sa}. \qquad (5.11.21)$$

Now, we can look for a solution of these equations in which $P_{sa}(t_j^+)$ and $P_{sa}(t_j^-)$ are independent of j. We express this by means of the notation

$$P_{sa}(t_j^+) = P_{sa}^+ \quad \text{(systolic pressure)} \qquad (5.11.22)$$

$$P_{sa}(t_j^-) = P_{sa}^- \quad \text{(diastolic pressure)}. \qquad (5.11.23)$$

Thus, P_{sa}^+ and P_{sa}^- satisfy

$$P_{sa}^- = P_{sa}^+ \Theta \qquad (5.11.24)$$

$$P_{sa}^+ = P_{sa}^- + \Delta V_o/C_{sa}. \qquad (5.11.25)$$

These are the same equations as (5.11.8) and (5.11.9) for the periodic systolic and diastolic pressures. This confirms that our theory of irregular arterial pulses contains the periodic pulse as a special case. (There are other solutions of (5.11.20) and (5.11.21) that do not correspond to a periodic pressure pulse even though the heartbeat and stroke volume are regular. Can you show that these solutions approach the periodic pulse as time increases?)

5.12   Annotated References

Many of the concepts used in this Chapter were pioneered by A.C. Guyton. See, for example:

Guyton A.C.: *Circulatory Physiology: Cardiac Output and its Regulation.* Saunders, Philadelphia, PA, 1963.

The idea that each cardiac ventricle can be modeled as a time-varying compliance and hence that the stroke volume can be determined from a pressure-volume loop (Fig. 5.5) comes from the work of K. Sagawa and his colleagues:

Sagawa, K., Suga, H. and Nakayama, K.: Instantaneous pressure-volume ratio of the left ventricle versus instantaneous force-length relation of papillary muscle. In: *Cardiovascular System Dynamics* (Baan, J., Noordergraaf, A., and Raines, J., eds.), M.I.T. Press, Cambridge, MA, 1978, 99–105.

Neural control of the circulation is discussed in the following references:

Karloff, et al.: Adaptation of the left ventricle to sudden changes in heart rate in patients with artificial pacemakers. *Cardiovascular Research*, **7**: 322, 1973.

Korner, P.I.: Integrative neural control of the circulation, *Physiological Reviews* **51**, 312–367, 1971.

Rowell, L.B.: Human cardiovascular adjustments to exercise and thermal stress, *Physiological Reviews*, **54**, 75–159, 1974.

Topham, W.S. and Warner, H.R.: The control of cardiac output during exercise. In: *Physical Bases of Circulatory Transport: Regulation and Exchange* (Reeve and Guyton, eds.), Saunders, Philadelphia, PA, 1967.

Our emphasis on oxygen as the key factor in autoregulation (Section 5.9) can be traced back to the work of Guyton:

Guyton, A.C., Ross, J.M., Carrier, O., Jr. and Walker, J.R.: Evidence for tissue oxygen demand as the major factor causing autoregulation, *Circulation Research*, **14**, 60, 1964.

The particular model of autoregulation that we use is simplified from:

Huntsman, L.L., Attinger, E.O., and Noordergraaf, A.: Metabolic autoregulation of blood flow in skeletal muscle: A model. In: *Cardiovascular System Dynamics* (Baan, J., Noordergraaf, A., and Raines, J., eds.), M.I.T. Press, Cambridge, MA, 1978, 400-414.

For a comprehensive discussion of the fetal circulation and the changes in the circulation occurring at birth, see the first few chapters of:

Rudolph, A.M.: *Congenital diseases of the heart*, Year Book Medical Publishers, Chicago, IL, 1974.

Rudolph's book is written in such a way that the mathematically inclined reader will find many opportunities for the construction of medically relevant mathematical models.

Finally, for a slightly more advanced look at some of the material presented in this Chapter, see:

Peskin, C.S.: Control of the heart and circulation, In: *Mathematical Aspects of Physiology* (Hoppensteadt, F.C., ed.), *Lectures in Applied Mathematics*, **19**, American Mathematical Society, Providence, RI, 1981, 1–38.

Exercises

5.1. CIRCULATION TIMES[2]

Given that the total blood volume is 5 liters and that the cardiac output is 5.6 liters/minute, calculate the time it takes for a "typical" red blood cell to go once around the circulation. This is called the *circulation time*.

First, consider the simplest possible model in which the circulation is a single loop and all cells take the same amount of time to traverse the loop.

Next, consider a more realistic model in which the circulation consists of several parallel loops with different circulation times. Let the volumes occupied by these loops be $V_1, \ldots, V_n$, let their blood flows be $Q_1, \ldots, Q_n$, and their circulation times be $T_1, \ldots, T_n$, respectively. Note that

$$V_o = V_1 + \ldots + V_n$$

and

$$Q = Q_1 + \ldots + Q_n.$$

Make up a reasonable definition of average circulation time and show that the result is the same as in the single loop case.

5.2. TABLE 5.2

Write out the formulae used to construct Table 5.2, and check that the numerical values in the table are correct.

5.3. PARAMETER CHANGES

Starting from the parameter values given in Table 5.2, find the effect of varying the parameters *one at a time*. Fill in Table 5.4:

Table 5.4. The Effect of Parameter Changes on the Uncontrolled Circulation

	Normal	K_r	K_L	R_s	R_p	V_o	units
		\multicolumn{5}{c}{50% Reduction In}				
Q	5.6						liters/min
P_{sa}	100						mm Hg
P_{sv}	2						mm Hg
P_{pa}	15						mm Hg
P_{pv}	5						mm Hg
V_{sa}	1.0						liters
V_{sv}	3.5						liters
V_{pa}	0.1						liters
V_{pv}	0.4						liters

---

[2]Warning: Exercise 5.1 is not related to the rest of the Chapter, and many students find it confusing. It should probably be skipped.

(In each case, the named parameter is reduced to half its normal value while all other parameters are held at their normal values.)

5.4. SENSITIVITY TO PARAMETER CHANGES

Transform Table 5.4. into a table of sensitivities. Note that all of the sensitivities fall in the range $-1 < \sigma < 1$.

5.5. DISCUSSION OF THE EFFECTS OF PARAMETER CHANGES

Discuss the results of Exercises 5.3 and 5.4. In particular, compare the effects of changing K_r with those of changing K_L, and compare the effects of changing R_s with those of changing R_p. Note the shifts in blood volume that accompany the changes in parameters and explain these shifts as best you can.

5.6. COMPARISON OF THE CONTROLLED AND UNCONTROLLED CIRCULATION BEHAVIOR

Make a graph that shows how cardiac output and systemic arterial pressure vary as functions of systemic resistance in the *uncontrolled* circulation. Consider the interval $0 < R_s < R_s^{normal}$. Construct a similar graph for the *controlled* circulation. (Use the same scales for the controlled and the uncontrolled cases.) Discuss the difference between the two cases.

5.7. UNCONTROLLED CIRCULATION: EFFECT OF A MORE REALISTIC COMPLIANCE EQUATION

This exercise and the next two develop some improvements in the model of the uncontrolled circulation. First, in each compliance vessel, replace the relation $V = C\,P$ by the more realistic formula $V = C\,P + V_d$. Show that the model remains the same as before, but that the volumes appearing in it must now be interpreted as excess volumes. Thus, our procedure for estimating C is no longer correct for the revised model. See Exercise 5.17.

5.8. UNCONTROLLED CIRCULATION: EFFECT OF NONZERO P_{thorax}

In our model of the uncontrolled circulation, we also neglected P_{thorax}. Fix this up by changing the equations of the right and left hearts and the pulmonary compliance to the following:

$$
\begin{aligned}
Q_r &= (FC_r)(P_{sv} - P_{thorax}) = K_r(P_{sv} - P_{thorax}) \\
Q_L &= (FC_L)(P_{pv} - P_{thorax}) = K_L(P_{pv} - P_{thorax}) \\
V_{pa} &= C_{pa}(P_{pa} - P_{thorax}) \\
V_{pv} &= C_{pv}(P_{pv} - P_{thorax}).
\end{aligned}
$$

Here P_{thorax} is a (negative) parameter and the volumes are understood to mean *excess* volumes as in the foregoing exercise. Solve the equations of the improved model and plot Q and P_{sv} as function of P_{thorax} for $P_{thorax} \leq 0$.

5.9. UNCONTROLLED CIRCULATION: EFFECT OF LOCALIZED PARTIAL VENOUS COLLAPSE

When P_{thorax} is sufficiently negative, P_{sv} becomes negative in the preceding exercise. This has the effect that the systemic veins experience partial collapse at the point where they enter the thorax. The partial collapse prevents P_{sv} from falling below zero, but it puts a (variable) resistance R_c between the systemic veins and the right atrium. In this situation, we have two additional unknowns: R_c = resistance of the partially collapsed veins, and P_{ra} = pressure in the right atrium. The additional equations are

$$P_{sv} = 0$$

$$Q_s R_c = P_{sv} - P_{ra} = 0 - P_{ra}.$$

Moreover, the equation of the right heart is replaced by

$$Q_r = (FC_r)(P_{ra} - P_{thorax}) = K_r(P_{ra} - P_{thorax})$$

in which P_{ra} replaces P_{sv}. (Note that the excess systemic venous volume is now zero, see Exercise 5.7. Thus, C_{sv} no longer plays any role in the model.)

Solve the equations of this revised model and show that Q is now independent of P_{thorax} and that R_c increases as P_{thorax} becomes more negative. Note that Q is also independent of K_r. (Warning: This solution only applies when P_{thorax} is sufficiently negative. At the transition value of P_{thorax}, $R_c = 0$.) Correct the graph of Exercise 5.8 by taking into account the results of this problem.

5.10. CALCULATION

Using the formula $P_{sa} = Q\,R_s$, derive the relationship

$$(-\sigma_{QR_s}) + \sigma_{P_{sa}R_s} = 1.$$

5.11. CONTROLLED CIRCULATION

In the model of the controlled circulation in Section 5.8 we assumed that the heart rate F is adjusted to achieve a certain target arterial pressure $P_{sa} = P^*$. There are patients in whom the heart rate cannot respond in this way. Then F is a fixed parameter. In these patients, however, the baroreceptor loop is still important because of its effects on the veins (see Figure 5.7). These effects were neglected in the model presented in Section 5.8, but they become very important when the heart rate is fixed.

Develop a model in which F is a parameter but C_{sv} is adjusted to achieve $P_{sa} = P^*$. Compare this model to the model of section 5.8. What are the similarities and differences of the two models with regard to their responses to changes in parameters? Consider changes in R_s and V_o and the responses of the cardiac output, the stroke volume, the heart rate, and the systemic arterial pressure.

Some patients have *pacemakers* in which the heart rate is an adjustable parameter that the patient can control by turning a knob with an external magnet. If such a patient increases his heart rate while he is *resting*, the cardiac output does not go up. Instead, the stroke volume falls. Does your model predict this? See what happens to cardiac output and stroke volume in your model when F changes while all of the other parameters are held constant.

5.12. Venous Oxygen as an Index of Blood Flow in Relation to Oxygen Consumption

Using Equation (5.9.2), plot $[O_2]_v/[O_2]_a$ as a function of $Q[O_2]_a/M$.

5.13. Autoregulation

Demonstrate the validity of the five characteristics of autoregulation that are listed at the end of section 5.9.

5.14. Fetal Circulation

In our discussion of the fetal circulation, we made no use of the compliance equations, so we could not solve the problem completely. We only determined the ratio of flows. Use the appropriate compliance equations and solve for Q, P_a, P_v, and the four volumes in the fetal case.

5.15. The State of the Circulation Immediately after Birth

In the equations of the fetal circulation, assume that $R_d = 0, K_r = K_L = K$ and $R_p < R_s$. This is roughly the situation just *after* birth with the ductus still open, the two sides of the heart still roughly equal, but with the lungs expanded and the blood flow to the placenta shut off. Show that the closed foramen solution is self-consistent in this case. Find a formula for Q_d and show that $Q_d < 0$.

5.16. Closure of the Ductus Arteriosus

Consider the situation described in exercise 5.15, but with $R_d \neq 0$ and with $K_r \neq K_L$. Solve for Q_d, Q_r, Q_L, P_{sa} and P_{pa} as functions of the parameters.

Fix all of the parameters except R_d at their normal adult values and plot these flows and pressures as functions of R_d. Plot all of the flows on one graph and the two pressures on another. (This shows roughly the changes that occur in the circulation as the ductus closes ($R_d \to \infty$) except, of course, that the other parameters may be changing and they are certainly not at their adult values.)

5.17. ESTIMATE OF ARTERIAL COMPLIANCE FROM THE ARTERIAL PULSE

The dynamics of the arterial pulse give us an alternative way to estimate C_{sa}. We have $\Delta V_o = C_{sa}\Delta P_{sa}$ where $\Delta V_o = 0.070$ liters is the stroke volume and where $\Delta P_{sa} = 40$ mm Hg is the pulse pressure. Calculate C_{sa} from these data.

Note that the result does not agree with the value of C_{sa} in Table 5.2 that was calculated from the formula $V_{sa} = C_{sa}P_{sa}$ using the normal resting (mean) values $< V_{su} > = 1$ liter and $< P_{sa} > = 100$ mm Hg.

A possible explanation of this discrepancy is that the equation $V_{sa} = C_{sa}P_{sa}$ is not a good approximation. Suppose we use $V_{sa} = C_{sa}P_{sa} + (V_d)_{sa}$, where $(V_d)_{sa}$ is constant. Then $\Delta V_{sa} = C_{sa}\Delta P_{sa}$, so the arterial compliance can be determined from the stroke volume and pulse pressure, as above. Once C_{sa} is known, we can use the mean arterial pressure and volume to determine $(V_d)_{sa}$ from the equation

$$(V_d)_{sa} = < V_{sa} > - C_{sa} < P_{sa} > .$$

Evaluate $(V_d)_{sa}$ in this way and make a graph showing the systemic arterial pressure as a function of volume. Mark the points corresponding to systolic and diastolic pressures on this plot when the blood pressure is 120/80.

5.18. MEAN ARTERIAL PRESSURE

Derive the formula for the mean arterial pressure (5.11.14) in two different ways:

1. by evaluating the integral (5.11.13) using the fact that that an exponential function is its own derivative

2. by evaluating the average of N equally spaced samples of $P_{sa}(t)$ and then taking the limit as $N \to \infty$. When evaluating the average, it is helpful to note that the samples of $P_{sa}(t)$ form a (finite) geometric sequence, since $P_{sa}(t)$ is exponential.

5.19. CALCULATION CONCERNING THE PERIODIC ARTERIAL PULSE

Using $R_s = 17.5$ mm Hg/(liter/min), $C_{sa} = 0.00175$ liters/mm Hg {see Exercise 5.17}, $\Delta V_o = 0.070$ liters and $T = (1/80)$ min. Evaluate $\Theta =$

$\exp(-T/(R_s C_{sa}))$ and then use Θ to evaluate the systolic pressure, the diastolic pressure, the pulse pressure, and the mean arterial pressure in the periodic case.

5.20. PULSE PRESSURE VERSUS MEAN ARTERIAL PRESSURE

Think of two different limiting cases in which the pulse pressure approaches zero while the mean arterial pressure and the cardiac output remain constant.

5.21. CIRCULATION DURING EXERCISE

During exercise in the model of the controlled circulation, R_s falls but T falls proportionally (heart rate goes up) and stroke volume is constant. Also, C_{sa} is constant. What happens to the systolic, diastolic and pulse pressures in this situation?

5.22. CIRCULATION DURING EXERCISE WITH THE HEART RATE FIXED

Suppose that a patient with a fixed heart rate performs exercise (so that R_s is reduced) and suppose she manages to raise her stroke volume enough so that her mean arterial pressure remains constant. What happens to the systolic, diastolic, and pulse pressures in this case?

5.23. CARDIAC ARREST

Suppose that a patient has suffered cardiac arrest for a long enough time that his arterial blood pressure is essentially zero. (Estimate how long this will take using the exponential decay of the arterial pressure in the absence of heartbeats. To be specific, what is the "half-life" of the arterial pressure as it decays in the absence of heartbeats?) Then his heart suddenly recovers. Make the unrealistic assumption that T, ΔV_o, R_s, and C_{sa} immediately assume their normal values as given in Exercise 5.19. Calculate the arterial systolic and diastolic pressures on the first 10 beats. Plot the results in graph form.

5.24. ARRHYTHMIA

Consider a patient who has an *arrhythmia* in which the heartbeats alternate so that

$$
\begin{aligned}
\Delta V_j &= \Delta V_1 & j \text{ odd} \\
&= \Delta V_2 & j \text{ even} \\
T_j &= T_1 & j \text{ odd} \\
&= T_2 & j \text{ even}
\end{aligned}
$$

(recall that T_j is the time interval *following* beat j). The arrhythmia is regular, so that her arterial pulse also repeats every other beat. Thus,

$$P(t_j^+) \quad = \quad P_1^+ \quad j \text{ odd}$$
$$= \quad P_2^+ \quad j \text{ even}$$

and

$$P(t_j^-) \quad = \quad P_1^- \quad j \text{ odd}$$
$$= \quad P_2^- \quad j \text{ even.}$$

Solve for P_1^+, P_2^+, P_1^-, and P_2^- as functions of the parameters ΔV_1, ΔV_2, T_1, T_2, R_s, and C_{sa}.

Check your solution for symmetry (it should be invariant when the subscripts 1 and 2 are interchanged). Also, check it by considering the special case where $\Delta V_1 = \Delta V_2$ and $T_1 = T_2$. What should happen to your solution then?

Plot the form of the pulse when T_1 and T_2 are such that $\Theta_1 = 2/3$, and $\Theta_2 = 1/2$ while $\Delta V_1 = 0.1$ liters and $\Delta V_2 = 0.05$ liters. (Note that the larger stroke volume comes after the larger filling period, since $T_2 > T_1$ and T_2 comes before ΔV_1.)

5.25. TWINS

Consider *hypothetical* twins who have the same values of R_s and C_{sa} and who both have abnormal rhythms that produce *identical* sequences of heart beats. This is, the times t_j and the stroke volumes ΔV_j are the same for both individuals although these sequences of times and stroke volumes are not at all regular.

At some time in the past, though, one of these individuals had an experience that shifted his blood pressure with respect to that of his twin. Write down the equations for each individual's blood pressure. Subtract these equations and show that their difference approaches zero exponentially with time.

6

Gas Exchange in the Lungs

The lungs contain about 3×10^8 *alveoli* (little sacs) in which air and blood are brought close together so that gas exchange can occur. The principal gases exchanged are O_2, which is picked up by the blood and CO_2, which leaves the blood stream and enters the air spaces of the lung. These gases need to cross the thin alveolar–capillary membrane; this occurs by diffusion. In normal circumstances, the alveolar–capillary membrane presents so slight a barrier to diffusion that the blood in the alveolar capillaries achieves *equilibrium* with the alveolar air before leaving the capillaries.

The blood leaving the right heart is subdivided many times by the branching pulmonary arterial tree before it reaches the alveoli. After passing through the alveoli, it is collected by the pulmonary veins. The alveolar capillaries are therefore connected *in parallel* in the sense that the pulmonary blood flow is the sum of the blood flows of the individual alveoli.

In a similar way, air entering the trachea is subdivided many times by the bronchial tree before it reaches the alveoli, and the total alveolar ventilation is the sum of the individual alveolar ventilations. Unlike the blood, however, the air leaves the alveoli on expiration by way of the same bronchial tree through which it entered on inspiration.

In this chapter, we discuss the laws that govern the transport of gases in the lung,[1], and we consider the conditions that lead to optimal transport of gases.

6.1 The Ideal Gas Law and the Solubility of Gases

The *ideal gas law* is approximately satisfied for many gases. This is stated as

$$P\,V = n\,k\,T \tag{6.1.1}$$

where
  P = pressure of the gas
  V = volume occupied by the gas
  n = number of molecules of the gas
  k = Boltzmann's constant

---

[1]Throughout this chapter, the phrase "the lung" is used to refer to the pulmonary tissue as a whole, which in fact is made up of two separate lungs.

T = absolute temperature.

Note that k is a universal constant which does not depend on the identity of the gas.[2] In a given volume at a given temperature, this law asserts that the pressure is proportional to the number of molecules. The physical reason for this is that the pressure is actually the force per unit area exerted by the molecules on the walls of the container as they collide with the walls and bounce back into the interior of the gas. If there are twice as many molecules, the pressure is twice as great.

In (6.1.1) the identity of the gas makes no difference. It does not matter, for example, whether the molecules are heavy or light. At a given temperature, the light molecules move faster and the force that they exert on the wall turns out to be the same as that of the heavy molecules. Only the *number* of molecules enters into the formula. This suggests that if we have a mixture of several ideal gases in a chamber, and if n_j is the number of molecules of gas j, then the pressure is given by the formula

$$PV = kT \sum n_j. \tag{6.1.2}$$

Let the *partial pressure* of the jth gas P_j be defined by

$$P_j V = n_j k T. \tag{6.1.3}$$

Then summing over j and comparing the result with (6.1.2), we see that

$$P = \sum P_j \tag{6.1.4}$$

so the total pressure is the sum of the partial pressures.

It is sometimes useful to relate the partial pressure of a gas to its concentration (i.e., the number of molecules per unit volume). The required formula is easily obtained by dividing both sides of (6.1.3) by V and letting $c_j = n_j/V$. The result is

$$P_j = c_j k T. \tag{6.1.5}$$

The concept of partial pressures can be extended to gases in solution. Consider the situation where a liquid and a gas are in contact across the surface of the liquid. Molecules of the gas can enter the liquid and wander for a time among its molecules; they are then said to be *dissolved* in the liquid, forming

---

[2]In the practical application of the ideal gas law, it is inconvenient that n, the number of molecules, is so large and that k, Boltzmann's constant, is so small. This is generally circumvented by multiplying and dividing by Avagadro's number $N_A \cong 6 \times 10^{23}$, which is the number of atoms in one gram of hydrogen. Thus, we get $PV = (n/N_A)(N_A k)T$. The constant $N_A k$ is called the "gas constant" and is usually denoted by R. The quantity n/N_A is called the number of "moles" and is usually denoted by n, but we shall use m to avoid confusion. Then the ideal gas law takes the form $PV = mRT$, in which the numbers that typically appear are less extreme than before. We shall use the form $PV = nkT$, however, because of its simpler physical interpretation: molecules are more fundamental than moles.

a *solution*. Molecules in solution can also leave the liquid at its surface and become part of the gas again.

After the system has been standing for a sufficiently long time, the rate at which gas molecules enter the solution becomes equal to the rate at which they leave. When this is true for all of the gases present, the system is said to be at *equilibrium*. If the gas molecules move independently of each other, it is not hard to see that the concentration of the gas in solution is proportional (at equilibrium) to its partial pressure in the gas. Solutions that obey this law are called *simple solutions*. For such solutions, we have

$$c_j = \sigma_j P_j \tag{6.1.6}$$

where c is the concentration, σ is the *solubility*, and P is the partial pressure. As before, the subscript j labels the gas. Of course, Equation (6.1.6) can be solved to yield

$$P_j = c_j / \sigma_j. \tag{6.1.7}$$

Given a simple solution in which the concentration of gas j is c_j, Equation (6.1.7) tells us the partial pressure of gas j that is needed to maintain this concentration if the solution is allowed to equilibrate with a gaseous phase. We summarize this by saying that the partial pressure of gas j in the *solution* is P_j.

These concepts can be extended to gases that do not form simple solutions. (An important example is O_2 in blood, see Section 6.6.) First, the linear relation (6.1.6) is replaced by a nonlinear relation

$$c_j = C_j(P_j) \tag{6.1.8}$$

in which C_j is an increasing function. Because C_j is increasing, it has an inverse function C_j^{-1} such that

$$P_j = C_j^{-1}(c_j). \tag{6.1.9}$$

Note that C_j^{-1} is also an increasing function. Equation (6.1.9) tells us the partial pressure that we need in a gaseous phase in contact with the liquid to maintain the concentration c_j. We call this the partial pressure of the gas in the liquid even when no gaseous phase is physically present.

Throughout most of this chapter we will consider gases that form simple solutions in blood. These include certain anesthetics that are cleared from the body by the lungs. Then in Section 6.6 we consider the transport of oxygen. Because oxygen is carried in blood by hemoglobin, its behavior is different from that of a simple solution.

6.2   The Equations of Gas Transport in One Alveolus

We consider the transport of one particular gas in the alveolus of Figure 6.1.

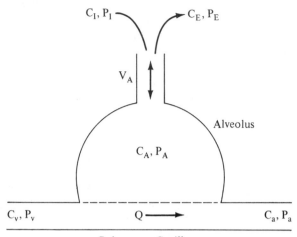

FIGURE 6.1.

Let

$$
\begin{aligned}
V_A &= \text{alveolar ventilation} \\
Q &= \text{blood flow} \\
c &= \text{concentration of the gas of interest} \\
P &= \text{partial pressure of the gas of interest} \\
\sigma &= \text{solubility of the gas of interest} \\
k &= \text{Boltzmann constant} \\
T &= \text{absolute temperature.}
\end{aligned}
$$

On the variables c and P, the subscripts I, A, E, v, and a have the following meanings:

$$
\begin{aligned}
I &= \text{inspired air} \\
A &= \text{alveolar air} \\
E &= \text{expired air} \\
v &= \text{venous blood} \\
a &= \text{arterial blood.}
\end{aligned}
$$

Several of the terms used in the foregoing require discussion.

The *alveolar ventilation* is the volume of fresh air delivered to the alveolus per unit time. This is equal to the product of the volume of fresh air brought in on each breath and the number of breaths per unit time. In this definition it is important that we specify *fresh* air, since the first part of the air that reaches the alveolus on each breath is simply the air that was expelled on the previous breath and remained in the bronchial tree between breaths. This *dead space* volume is not included in the alveolar ventilation. Strictly speaking, we should distinguish between the alveolar ventilation of inspiration and the alveolar ventilation of expiration. These are not quite equal because the consumption of O_2 by the body is not exactly equal to the production of CO_2. This distinction will be ignored here, and we therefore need only one quantity, V_A, the alveolar ventilation.

By *venous blood* we mean the blood entering the alveolus, despite the fact that this blood flows in vessels that are part of the pulmonary arterial tree. the reason for this designation is that the chemical composition of this blood is identical to that in the systemic veins. In particular, the venous blood is relatively depleted of O_2 and relatively rich in CO_2. By arterial blood we mean the blood leaving the alveolus, which is relatively rich in O_2 and relatively free of CO_2 and which is destined to become the systemic arterial blood. Again, this designation ignores the fact that this arterial blood flows in the pulmonary veins. Thus, we name the blood according to its chemical composition instead of the type of vessels through which it travels.

To derive the equations of gas transport in one alveolus, we make the following assumptions:

1. Steady state. The number of molecules of the gas of interest entering the alveolus per unit time is equal to the number of molecules leaving per unit time. Note that molecules may enter by the air or blood and they may also leave by the air or blood. This can be summarized by an equation that describes the conservation of molecules:

$$V_A c_I + Q\, c_v = V_A c_E + Q\, c_a. \qquad (6.2.1)$$

2. Expired air is a sample of alveolar air. Thus,

$$c_E = c_A. \qquad (6.2.2)$$

3. Ideal gas law. The gas of interest behaves like an ideal gas in the alveolar air:

$$P_A = k\, T\, c_A. \qquad (6.2.3)$$

4. Simple solution. The gas of interest forms a simple solution in blood. In particular, in the arterial blood

$$\sigma P_a = c_a. \qquad (6.2.4)$$

5. Equilibrium. As the blood passes through the alveolus, it achieves equilibrium with alveolar air. Thus, the partial pressure of each gas in the blood leaving the alveolus is the same as in the alveolar air:

$$P_a = P_A. \qquad (6.2.5)$$

The first two equations can be combined to yield

$$V_A(c_I - c_A) = Q\,(c_a - c_v).\tag{6.2.6}$$

The quantity on the left side of (6.2.6) represents the number of molecules of gas per unit time that are given up by the air; the quantity on the right represents the number of molecules of the gas picked up per unit time by the blood. In the steady state, these must be equal. Either side of (6.2.6) is therefore an expression for the net transport of the gas of interest in the alveolus. This immediately tells us something important (and perhaps surprising): For net transport of gas to occur, it is necessary that alveolar air have a different composition than inspired air $(c_I \neq c_A)$. For example, the partial pressure of O_2 in the inspired air is about 160 mm Hg whereas in the alveolus it is about 100 mm Hg. (The concentrations are proportional to partial pressures.) The partial pressure of CO_2 in the inspired air is essentially zero, whereas in the alveolus it is about 40 mm Hg.

Note that the sign of $c_I - c_A$ is positive for O_2 and negative for CO_2. This reflects the fact that the direction of gas transport is inward for O_2 and outward for CO_2.

Equations (6.2.3) through (6.2.5) can be combined to yield

$$c_a = \sigma k\, T\, c_A.\tag{6.2.7}$$

We now look on (6.2.6) and (6.2.7) as a pair of simultaneous equations in the two unknowns c_a and c_A. The solution is

$$\begin{aligned}
c_A &= [V_A c_I + Q c_v]/[V_A + Q\sigma\,k\,T]\\
&= [r c_I + c_v]/[r + \sigma k\,T]
\end{aligned}\tag{6.2.8}$$

$$c_a = \sigma\,k\,T\,[r c_I + c_v]/[r + \sigma kT]\tag{6.2.9}$$

where

$$r = V_A/Q.\tag{6.2.10}$$

It is an important fact that the compositions of the alveolar air and the arterial blood are determined not by the ventilation and blood flow separately, but only by the *ventilation–perfusion ratio* r. As $r \to \infty$, the composition of the alveolar air approaches that of the inspired air, since

$$\begin{aligned}
c_A &= [r c_I + c_v]/[r + \sigma\,k\,T]\\
&= [c_I + c_v/r]/[1 + \sigma\,k\,T/r]\\
&\to c_I \text{ as } r \to \infty,
\end{aligned}\tag{6.2.11}$$

and the composition of arterial blood approaches equilibrium with inspired air. As $r \to 0$, $c_A \to c_v/\sigma kT$, so the composition of arterial blood $c_a = \sigma kT c_A$ approaches that of the venous blood. In this limit, the composition of alveolar air approaches equilibrium with the venous blood. In fact, the ventilation–perfusion ratio is not too different from unity, and the alveolar and arterial

partial pressures are between the corresponding inspired and venous partial
pressures.

We now derive a formula for the net transport of the gas of interest. As
mentioned above, this is given by the right- or by the left-hand side of (6.2.6).
Using the right-hand side and substituting the formula for c_a, (6.2.9), we get

$$
\begin{aligned}
f &= Q(c_a - c_v) \\
&= Qr(\sigma kTc_I - c_v)/(r + \sigma kT) \\
&= (P_I - P_v)Qr\sigma/[r + \sigma kT]
\end{aligned}
\tag{6.2.12}
$$

where we have used $P_I = kTc_I$ and $\sigma P_v = c_v$. The reader should verify that
the same result is obtained if we start from $f = V_A(c_I - c_A)$ and use the
formula for c_A, (6.2.8).

The formula (6.2.12) for the flux of gas has the following simple interpretation. The quantity $Q\sigma(P_I - P_v)$ is the flux of gas that would occur if the
venous blood were allowed to equilibrate directly with inspired air. To get the
actual flux, we multiply this by the fraction $r/[r + \sigma kT]$, which involves the
ventilation–perfusion ratio, r.

6.3   Gas Transport in the Lung

We now take account of the fact that the lung consists of some 3×10^8 alveoli
connected in parallel. Several of the physical quantities that appear in the
previous section have the same value in all of the different alveoli of the lung.
Because the inflowing venous blood is simply partitioned among the various
alveoli, its composition is constant throughout the lung. For the same reason,
the composition of the inspired air is the same for all of the different alveoli.
The solubility of any gas in blood is the same in different parts of the lung.
The Boltzmann constant certainly does not vary, and we make the assumption
that the temperature is uniform throughout the lung.

The ventilation V_A and the perfusion Q can certainly differ in different
alveoli. Because of the effects of gravity, there is a systematic gradient of
perfusion in the lung: The lower parts have a substantially larger blood flow
than the upper parts of the lung. This is caused by the effects of hydrostatic
pressure on the freely distensible pulmonary vessels. The ventilation is also
greater in the lower parts of the lung. To understand this, recall that alveolar
ventilation depends on the *difference* between the maximum and minimum
volume of the alveolus during the breathing cycle. The maximum volumes
achieved during inspiration are fairly uniform throughout the lung, but the
minimum volumes achieved during expiration are smaller in the lower part of
the lung because the weight of the lung tissue participates in the compression
of the alveoli. Accordingly, the alveolar ventilation, like the blood flow, is
larger in the lower parts of the lung. These effects do not exactly balance,
however, so the ratio of ventilation to perfusion is different in different alveoli.

More extreme variations in the ratio of ventilation to perfusion occur in
pulmonary disease. Either the air supply or the blood supply to an alveolus

can be completely obliterated resulting in a ventilation–perfusion ratio of zero or infinity.

Thus, we cannot regard the ventilation–perfusion ratio as constant. From equations (6.2.8) and (6.2.9), it is clear that variations in r, the ratio of ventilation to perfusion, will result in variations in the composition of the alveolar air and of the blood leaving the alveolus. From (6.2.12), it is clear that the flux of gas is also different in alveoli with different values of r.

To analyze the situation in which the ventilation–perfusion ratio may vary, we number the alveoli using an index $i, i = 1, \ldots, 3 \times 10^8$. Quantities that do not vary from one alveolus to the next are written without the index i. Accordingly, we have

$$(c_A)_i = (r_i c_I + c_v)/(r_i + \sigma kT) \tag{6.3.1}$$

$$(c_a)_i = \sigma kT(r_i c_I + c_v)/(r_i + \sigma kT) \tag{6.3.2}$$

where

$$r_i = (V_A)_i/Q_i \tag{6.3.3}$$

and the flux of gas in the ith alveolus is given by

$$f_i = Q_i r_i \sigma(P_I - P_v)/[r_i + \sigma kT]. \tag{6.3.4}$$

By summing (6.3.4) over all the alveoli, we derive an equation for the transport of the gas of interest in the lung as a whole. The formula is

$$f = \Sigma_i f_i = \sigma(P_I - P_V)\Sigma Q_i r_i/[r_i + \sigma kT]. \tag{6.3.5}$$

Multiplying and dividing by the total pulmonary blood flow, we find that f can be written in the form

$$f = \sigma(P_I - P_v)Q_o E \tag{6.3.6}$$

where

$$E = (1/Q_o)\Sigma_i Q_i r_i/[r_i + \sigma kT] \tag{6.3.7}$$

$$Q_o = \Sigma_i Q_i. \tag{6.3.8}$$

As in the case of a single alveolus, we remark that $\sigma(P_I - P_v)Q_o$ is the transport that would occur if venous blood were brought directly into contact with room air. The quantity E is a fraction $(0 < E < 1)$ that can be thought of as the *efficiency* of gas transport.

6.4   Optimal Gas Transport

Suppose we are given the total alveolar ventilation

$$(V_A)_o = \Sigma_i (V_A)_i \tag{6.4.1}$$

and the total pulmonary blood flow

$$Q_o = \Sigma_i Q_i. \tag{6.4.2}$$

How should this airflow and blood flow be distributed to maximize the magnitude of f for given P_I and P_v? Alternatively, we could ask how the airflow and blood flow should be distributed to minimize the magnitude of $P_I - P_v$ for given f? The first problem is appropriate when the rate of transport is determined by the lung, as in the case of anesthetic gases that are cleared from the body by the lungs. The second problem is appropriate for gases like O_2 and CO_2, for which the rate of transport is fixed by the tissues. For such a gas, the venous partial pressure automatically adjusts to whatever value is needed to maintain adequate flux across the lung. In any case, it is clear from (6.3.6) that we can solve both problems simultaneously by maximizing the efficiency

$$E = (1/Q_o)\Sigma_i Q_i r_i / [r_i + \sigma kT]. \tag{6.4.3}$$

We now show that

$$E \le E_{\max} \tag{6.4.4}$$

where

$$
\begin{aligned}
E_{\max} &= (1/Q_o)\Sigma_i Q_i r_o / [r_o + \sigma kT] \\
&= r_o / [r_o + \sigma kT]
\end{aligned}
\tag{6.4.5}
$$

and

$$r_o = (V_A)_o / Q_o. \tag{6.4.6}$$

Note that r_o is the ventilation–perfusion ratio for the lung as a whole and that $E_{\max}$ is the efficiency of gas transport when the ventilation–perfusion ratio of each alveolus matches that of the lung as a whole. Our goal is to prove that the efficiency of gas transport cannot be greater than $E_{\max}$. (The efficiency $E_{\max}$ is actually achieved by setting $r_i = r_o$ for all i.)

To prove this, we use the fact that the function

$$g(r) = r/[r + \sigma kT] \tag{6.4.7}$$

lies below all of its tangent lines (see Figure 6.2). This can be shown by taking the second derivative (curvature) of g, which is

$$g''(r) = -2\sigma kT/[r + \sigma kT]^3 < 0. \tag{6.4.8}$$

It follows that

$$g(r_i) \le g(r_o) + (r_i - r_o)g'(r_o). \tag{6.4.9}$$

(This inequality just expresses the fact that the function lies below the line that is tangent to g at r_o.) Now, we use (6.4.9) to derive a bound on E as follows:

$$Q_o E = \Sigma_i Q_i g(r_i) \le \Sigma_i Q_i g(r_o) + \Sigma_i Q_i (r_i - r_o)g'(r_o). \tag{6.4.10}$$

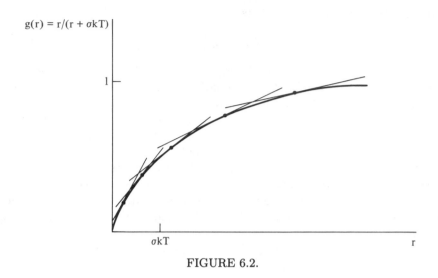

$g(r) = r/(r + \sigma kT)$

σkT

r

FIGURE 6.2.

Using the constraints and the definitions of r_i and r_o, the reader can show that the last term on the right is zero {see Exercise 6.2} Thus,

$$Q_o E \leq \Sigma_i Q_i g(r_o) = Q_o E_{\max} \qquad (6.4.11)$$

so

$$E \leq E_{\max} \qquad (6.4.12)$$

as promised.

We have shown that optimal gas transport is achieved when the *ventilation–perfusion ratio* is constant throughout the lung. Note that the separate distributions of airflow and blood flow are not important, as long as these distributions are *matched* in the sense that their ratio is constant.

6.5   Mean Alveolar and Arterial Partial Pressures

We have just seen that inhomogeneity of the ventilation–perfusion ratio degrades the efficiency of gas transport. Another manifestation of the same phenomenon is the lack of equilibrium between alveolar air and arterial blood that occurs as a result of nonuniform ventilation–perfusion ratio. The "alveolar air" mentioned in the foregoing is the air that is expelled from the whole population of pulmonary alveoli during exhalation. Note that this is a mixture of air samples from the different alveoli; accordingly, we refer to it as the *mixed alveolar air*. Each alveolus contributes to this mixture in proportion to its own alveolar ventilation. Similarly, the (systemic) arterial blood is a mixture obtained by combining the streams of blood flowing through the pulmonary capillaries of the various alveoli. The contribution of each alveolus to the *mixed* (systemic) *arterial blood* is proportional to the blood flow (perfusion) of the alveolus in question.

The following argument seems to prove that mixed alveolar air and mixed arterial blood are in equilibrium. In each alveolus, the expired air and the blood leaving the alveolus are in equilibrium. Accordingly, the mixed alveolar air must be in equilibrium with the mixed arterial blood. This argument is incorrect, and the mean alveolar partial pressure is not necessarily equal to the mean arterial blood pressure, as we now show.

The *mean arterial concentration* of the gas of interest, $< c_a >$, is calculated as follows:

$$< c_a >= [\Sigma_i Q_i (c_a)_i]/Q_o. \tag{6.5.1}$$

The numerator of this fraction is the number of molecules of the gas of interest entering the arterial blood from the alveoli per unit of time. The mean arterial partial pressure of the gas is computed from $< c_a >$ as follows:

$$< P_a >=< c_a > /\sigma = [\Sigma_i Q_i (c_a)_i]/Q_o \sigma \tag{6.5.2}$$

where σ is the solubility of the gas in blood.

Since expired air is a sample of alveolar air, we define the mean alveolar concentration in terms of the expired air:

$$< c_A >= [\Sigma_i (V_A)_i (c_A)_i]/(V_A)_o. \tag{6.5.3}$$

The mean alveolar partial pressure is then given by

$$< P_A >= kT < c_A >= kT[\Sigma_i (V_A)_i (c_A)_i]/(V_A)_o. \tag{6.5.4}$$

Using equations (6.3.1) through (6.3.3) and (6.4.6), we get

$$< P_A >= (kT/Q_o)\Sigma_i Q_i (r_i/r_o)(r_i c_I + c_v)/(r_i + \sigma kT) \tag{6.5.5}$$

$$< P_a >= (kT/Q_o)\Sigma_i Q_i (r_i c_I + c_v)/(r_i + \sigma kT). \tag{6.5.6}$$

Subtracting these equations gives

$$< P_A > - < P_a >= (kT/(r_o Q_o))\Sigma_i Q_i (r_i - r_o)(r_i c_I + c_v)/(r_i + \sigma kT). \tag{6.5.7}$$

But,

$$[r_i c_I + c_v]/[r_i + \sigma kT] = [r_o c_I + c_v]/[r_o + \sigma kT] \tag{6.5.8}$$
$$+(r_i - r_o)[\sigma kT c_I - c_v]/[(r_i + \sigma kT)(r_o + \sigma kT)].$$

Substituting (6.5.8) in (6.5.7) and using the fact that

$$\Sigma_i Q_i (r_i - r_o) = 0,$$

{see Exercise 6.2}, we get

$$< P_A > - < P_a > \tag{6.5.9}$$

$$= [\sigma kT(P_I - P_v)/((r_o + \sigma kT)(Q_o r_o))]\Sigma_i (r_i - r_o)^2 Q_i/[r_i + \sigma kT].$$

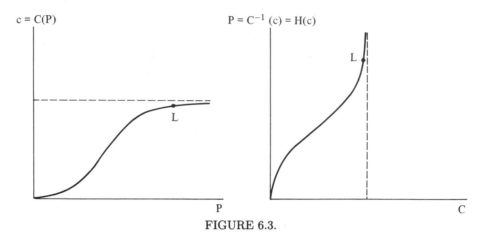

FIGURE 6.3.

Note that

$$\Sigma_i (r_i - r_o)^2 Q_i / [r_i + \sigma kT] \geq 0 \qquad (6.5.10)$$

with equality only when $r_i = r_o$ for all i. The condition $r_i = r_o$ for all i means that the ventilation–perfusion ratio is constant throughout the lung.

With these calculations, we have shown that mixed alveolar air and mixed arterial blood are in equilibrium ($< P_A >=< P_a >$) only if the ventilation–perfusion ratio is uniform throughout the lung. Otherwise, $< P_A > - < P_a >$ has the same sign as $P_I - P_v$. Since the latter quantity determines the direction of gas transport (see Equation 6.3.5), we conclude that for any gas transported into the body, $< P_A > \geq < P_a >$ with equality only for a homogeneous lung and that for any gas transported out of the body, $< P_A > \leq < P_a >$ with equality only for a homogeneous lung.

Thus, a nonuniform distribution of ventilation in relation to perfusion creates an effective barrier between air and blood, even when there is no such barrier in each individual alveolus. The practical consequence of such nonuniformity in the ventilation–perfusion ratio is that the body must increase the total ventilation, the cardiac output, or both in order to achieve normal levels of gas transport at normal partial pressures.

6.6   Transport of O_2

As mentioned in Section 6.1, O_2 does not form a simple solution in blood. The relation between partial pressure and concentration of O_2 in blood is plotted in Figure 6.3 in two ways: concentration as a function of partial and partial pressure as a function concentration. In this section, we use the latter relation

$$P = C^{-1}(c) = H(c) \qquad (6.6.1)$$

and we note that the function $H = C^{-1}$ has the following properties:

$$H(0) = 0 \qquad (6.6.2)$$

$$H'(c) > 0 \qquad (6.6.3)$$

where H' denotes the derivative of H with respect to c, and also, in the range of partial pressures that are relevant for the lung,

$$H''(c) > 0. \qquad (6.6.4)$$

In Section 6.2, the equations of gas transport in an alveolus were reduced to a pair of simultaneous equations for c_a and c_A. The corresponding equations for the case of O_2 are

$$r(c_I - c_A) = c_a - c_v \qquad (6.6.5)$$

$$kTc_A = H(c_a). \qquad (6.6.6)$$

Substituting (6.6.6) into (6.6.5), we get a nonlinear equation for c_a:

$$r(c_I - (1/kT)H(c_a)) = c_a - c_v \qquad (6.6.7)$$

or

$$r\,c_I + c_v = c_a + (r/kT)H(c_a). \qquad (6.6.8)$$

The expression on the left in (6.6.8) is a positive constant (for fixed r). As a function of c_a, the expression on the right is monotone increasing. It has the value zero at $c_a = 0$, and it increases without bound as $c_a \to \infty$. It follows that (6.6.8) has a unique solution c_a for each r. The solution depends on r, so we denote it as a function $c_a(r)$. It is important to note that this function is the same in all of the different alveoli on the lung. (The value of r, of course, can be different in different alveoli and so the value of c_a can also be different, but the function as a whole is the same for all alveoli of the lung.)

Although we cannot find the function $c_a(r)$ explicitly, we can find some of its properties. For instance, putting $r = 0$ in 6.6.8, we find that

$$c_a(0) = c_v. \qquad (6.6.9)$$

Putting $r = \infty$, we find

$$kT\,c_I = H(c_a(\infty)) \qquad (6.6.10)$$

which asserts that arterial blood is in equilibrium with inspired air at $r = \infty$.

Differentiating (6.6.7) twice with respect to r, we get

$$c_I - (1/kT)H(c_a) - (r/kT)H'(c_a)c_a' = c_a' \qquad (6.6.11)$$

$$-(2/kT)H'(c_a)c_a' - (r/kT)[H'(c_a)c_a'' + H''(c_a)(c_a')^2] = c_a''. \qquad (6.6.12)$$

Solving for c_a' and c_a'' and using (6.6.7) gives

$$c_a' = [c_I - (1/kT)H(c_a)]/[1 + (r/kT)H'(c_a)]$$

$$\qquad (6.6.13)$$

$$= [c_a - c_v]/[r(1 + (r/kT)H'(c_a))]$$

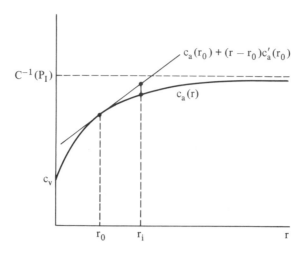

FIGURE 6.4.

$$c_a'' = -[(2/kT)H'(c_a)c_a'$$
$$+ (r/kT)H''(c_a)(c_a')^2]/[1 + (r/kT)H'(c_a)] \qquad (6.6.14)$$

Since O_2 is transported into the body, $c_a > c_v$. It follows from the properties of H listed above (6.6.2–6.6.3) that

$$c_a' > 0 \qquad (6.6.15)$$

$$c_a'' < 0. \qquad (6.6.16)$$

The function $c_a(r)$ is sketched in Figure 6.4.

The meaning of these results is as follows. The inequality $c_a' > 0$ means that the arterial oxygen concentration increases with increasing values of the ventilation–perfusion ratio. The inequality $c_a'' < 0$, on the other hand, means that the rate of increase diminishes as the ventilation–perfusion ratio is raised.

We are now ready to consider O_2 transport for the lung as a whole. The flow of O_2 is given by

$$f = \Sigma_i Q_i(c_a(r_i) - c_v). \qquad (6.6.17)$$

We shall prove that

$$f \le f_o = \Sigma_i Q_i(c_a(r_o) - c_v) \qquad (6.6.18)$$

where as before $r_i = (V_A)_i/Q_i$ and

$$r_o = (V_A)_o/Q_o$$
$$= \Sigma_i(V_A)_i/\Sigma_i Q_i. \qquad (6.6.19)$$

The proof is the same as for gases that form simple solutions. We have already shown that $c_a'' < 0$. It follows that c_a lies below its tangent lines. In particular,

$$c_a(r_i) \le c_a(r_o) + (r_i - r_o)c_a'(r_o). \qquad (6.6.20)$$

Multiplying by Q_i and summing, we get

$$\Sigma_i Q_i c_a(r_i) \leq \Sigma_i Q_i c_a(r_o) + c_a'(r_o)\Sigma_i Q_i(r_i - r_o). \qquad (6.6.21)$$

The last term is zero {see Exercise 6.2}, so we can subtract $c_v Q_o$ from both sides to get

$$f \leq f_o \qquad (6.6.22)$$

as required.

The inequality $f \leq f_o$ can be given two different interpretations depending on what we regard as given. If we are given c_I and c_v, then the flux of O_2 is determined by the lung and $f \leq f_o$ is a restriction on how big this flux can be.

Suppose, instead, that we are given c_I and f. This is the physiological situation since f is really determined by the tissues and since the venous O_2 concentration adjusts itself accordingly. Then the inequality $f \leq f_o$ can be reinterpreted as a restriction on c_v. To see what form this restriction takes, we have to make explicit the dependence of c_a on c_v. Thus, we replace the function $c_a(r)$ by $c_a(r, c_v)$. This function is defined as the solution of (6.6.8) from which it follows that ca increases as c_v increases with r fixed. From (6.6.7), though, we see that $c_a - c_v$ *decreases* as c_v (and so c_a) increases with r fixed. Let

$$\Delta_o(c_v) = c_a(r_o, c_v) - c_v. \qquad (6.6.23)$$

We have just shown that Δ_o is a decreasing function. Our inequality $f \leq f_o$ can be rewritten in terms of Δ_o as follows

$$f \leq Q_o \Delta_o(c_v). \qquad (6.6.24)$$

Let c_v^o be defined by the equation

$$f = Q_o \Delta_o(c_v^o). \qquad (6.6.25)$$

Thus, c_v^o is the venous oxygen concentration (for given f) when the ventilation–perfusion ratio is uniform throughout the lung. Combining (6.6.24) and (6.6.25), we see that

$$\Delta_o(c_v^o) \leq \Delta_o(c_v). \qquad (6.6.26)$$

Since Δ_o is decreasing, this implies that

$$c_v \leq c_v^o. \qquad (6.6.27)$$

That is, for a given rate of O_2 consumption by the body, the venous O_2 concentration is maximized when the ventilation–perfusion ratio is uniform throughout the lung. This is of importance because the systemic veins are in equilibrium with the tissues of the body. Thus, a high c_v means that oxygen is plentiful and that the performance of the various tissues is not limited by the oxygen supply.

6.7   Annotated References

This Chapter is strongly influenced by the following book, which emphasizes the importance of the ratio of ventilation to perfusion:

West, J.B.: *Ventilation/Blood Flow and Gas Exchange*, Blackwell, Oxford, UK, 1965.

The following paper also addresses the specific issue of optimal gas transport, which is the dominant theme of this Chapter:

Evans, J.W., Wagner, and West, J.B.: Conditions for reduction of pulmonary gas transfer by ventilation–perfusion inequality. *Journal of Applied Physiology*, **36**, 535–567, 1974.

Exercises

6.1. CALCULATION

Verify that (6.2.12) can also be derived starting from the formula

$$f = (V_A)(c_I - c_A).$$

6.2. CALCULATION

Show that

$$\Sigma_i Q_i(r_i - r_o) = 0$$

where $r_i = (V_A)_i/Q_i$ and $r_o = \Sigma_i(V_A)_i/\Sigma_i Q_i$.

6.3. REDUCTION OF ALVEOLAR POPULATION TO A SINGLE EFFECTIVE ALVEOLUS

Consider a collection of alveoli that all have the same ratio of ventilation to perfusion. Show that the whole collection is functionally equivalent to a single alveolus.

6.4. AN EXTREME MISMATCH OF VENTILATION AND PERFUSION

Consider a lung with two parts. In each part, the ventilation–perfusion ratio is constant. Suppose that the airflow and blood flow are as follows:

$$(V_A)_1 = 5.0 \text{ liters/min}, \quad Q_1 = 0.0 \text{ liters/min}$$
$$(V_A)_2 = 0.0 \text{ liters/min}, \quad Q_2 = 5.0 \text{ liters/min}$$

Calculate f, $< P_A >$ and $< P_a >$ in terms of P_I, P_v, σ, and kT. Explain your results in words.

6.5. OPTIMAL GAS TRANSPORT IN A TWO-COMPARTMENT LUNG

Consider a lung with two parts where in each part the ventilation–perfusion ratio is constant. Assume that $P_I = 0$, $\sigma kT = 1$, $Q_1 = 2.0$ liters/min, $Q_2 = 3.0$ liters/min, and $(V_A)_o = (V_A)_1 + (V_A)_2 = 5.0$ liters/min.

1. Find a formula for E as a function of $(V_A)_1$. Note that $(V_A)_2 = (V_A)_o - (V_A)_1$.

2. Determine the value of $(V_A)_1$ that maximizes E by setting $dE/d(V_A)_1 = 0$. Interpret your result in terms of ventilation/perfusion ratios.

3. Evaluate E_{max}, the value of E when $(V_A)_1$ has the optimal value determined above.

4. Plot E, $< P_a > /P_v$, $< P_A > /P_v$ as functions of $(V_A)_1$ over the interval $0 < (V_A)_1 < 5.0$. The mean partial pressures should both be plotted on the same graph. Explain how these graphs illustrate the theory of this chapter.

6.6. ARTERIAL O_2 SATURATION AS A FUNCTION OF r

There is a simple model of the interaction between O_2 and *hemoglobin* that predicts that the concentration of O_2 in blood is related to its partial pressure according to the formula

$$c = C(P) = c^* P^4 / [P_{1/2}^4 + P^4]$$

where c^* and $P_{1/2}$ are constants.

1. Solve this equation to obtain $P = H(c)$.

2. Divide equation (6.6.8) by c^* to obtain

$$r(c_I/c^*) + (c_v/c^*) = (c_a/c^*) + (r\ H(c_a)/kTc^*).$$

Assume that $c_I = c^*, c_v = 0.4c^*, kTc^* = 150$ mm Hg, and $P_{1/2} = 25$ mm Hg. Solve for c_a/c^* when $r = 0, \frac{1}{4}, \frac{1}{2}, 1, 2, 4, \infty$, and plot your results as a graph of c_a/c^* as a function of r. The solution has to be obtained by some approximation method. For example, fix r and plot the right-hand side as a function of c_a. The solution is the value of c_a where the right-hand side crosses the (constant) left-hand side. Whatever solution method you use, it has to be carried out separately for each of the values of r that are listed above.

7

Control of Cell Volume and the Electrical Properties of Cell Membranes

Cell contain proteins, nucleic acids, and other macromolecules that often carry many negative charges per molecule. This electrical charge is balanced by positive ions (especially potassium, denoted by K^+) that are dissolved in the intracellular water. These ions tend to draw water into the cells by osmosis, and the cells would swell and eventually burst if this osmotic effect were not offset by other factors.

The thick cell wall of plant cells can withstand considerable hydrostatic pressure, and an equilibrium is achieved in which the elevated pressure in the interior of the cell balances the osmotic effect.

Animal cells lack a cell wall, and their thin membranes cannot withstand any measurable pressure difference. Therefore, a more subtle mechanism is required to control cell volume. As we shall see, a by-product of this mechanism is that the membranes become charged. In a spectacular example of evolutionary spin-off, this electrical potential difference is used by nerve and muscle cells as a signaling mechanism.

7.1 Osmotic Pressure and the Work of Concentration

In Figure 7.1A, two chambers filled with water are separated by a rigid membrane. The pores make it possible for water to flow from one compartment to the other. Each compartment is equipped with a piston that can be used to apply pressure to that compartment and push water through the pores.

The volume rate of flow through the membrane is linearly related to the applied pressure difference as shown in Figure 7.1B. Thus, the flow Q is given by the simple equation

$$P_1 - P_2 = R\,Q \tag{7.1.1}$$

where R is the *flow resistance* of the membrane.

Now suppose that sugar is added to the compartment on the left, as in Figure 7.1C, and that the sugar molecules are too large to get through the pores in the membrane. The pressure–flow relation is now shifted from the

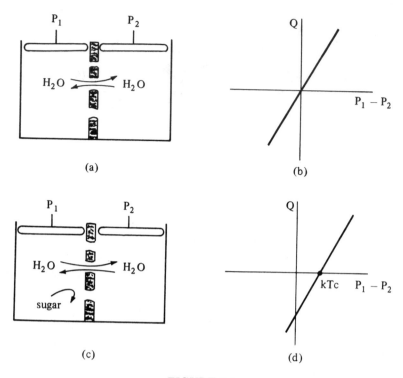

FIGURE 7.1.

origin, as shown in Figure 7.1D, so that the flow Q is now given by

$$P_1 - P_2 - kTc = R\,Q \qquad (7.1.2)$$

where c is the concentration of sugar, measured in molecules per unit volume.

According to Equation (7.1.2), a pressure difference given by $P_1 - P_2 = kTc$ must be applied merely to prevent the water from flowing from right to left into the sugar solution. If no such pressure difference is applied (i.e., $P_1 = P_2$), then the flow Q is given by $Q = -kTc/R$, as though a pressure difference equal to $-kTc$ had been applied in the absence of the sugar solution. The pressure kTc is called the *osmotic pressure*. Note that it tends to draw water into the compartment containing the sugar solution. If we write $c = n/V_1$, where n is the number of sugar molecules and V_1 is the volume in which they are distributed, then we see that

$$P_{osmotic} = kTc = nkT/V_1 \qquad (7.1.3)$$

so that the osmotic pressure is given by a formula that is identical to the ideal gas law!

What does an ideal gas have in common with a sugar solution? A gas is *ideal* if the interactions between its molecules can be neglected. The internal energy of an ideal gas is entirely kinetic (i.e., there is no energy of interaction between molecules). Similarly, in a (dilute) solution, the solute molecules wander around independently of each other. They can interact with the solvent, but only rarely do they encounter each other.

We now use these ideas to derive the formula (7.1.2) from energetic arguments. The assumptions are:

1. When the volume rate of flow through the membrane is Q, the rate at which work is *performed* by the pistons is given by

$$dW_{piston}/dt = (P_1 - P_2)\,Q \qquad (7.1.4)$$

{See Ex. 7.1}

2. The rate at which work is *required* to drive water through the pores in the membrane at the volume rate of flow Q is

$$dW_{membrane}/dt = R\,Q^2 \qquad (7.1.5)$$

3. The rate at which work is *required* to concentrate the sugar solution is the same as if the solute molecules were an ideal gas consisting of n molecules distributed in the volume V_1. In that case, we would have $P\,V_1 = n\,k\,T$, or simply $P = k\,T\,c$, since $c = n/V_1$. The work of concentration would be given by

$$\begin{aligned} dW_{concentration}/dt &= -PdV_1/dt \\ &= -kTc\,dV_1/dt. \end{aligned} \qquad (7.1.6)$$

We assume that this formula holds for a sugar solution as well as for an ideal gas. Since the flow through the membrane Q decreases the volume of solution on side 1 at the rate $dV_1/dt = -Q$, we have

$$dW_{concentration}/dt = kTc\,Q. \qquad (7.1.7)$$

4. Finally, by conservation of energy

$$dW_{piston}/dt = dW_{membrane}/dt + dW_{concentration}/dt. \qquad (7.1.8)$$

Substituting in 7.1.8 and dividing by Q, we obtain

$$(P_1 - P_2) = R\,Q + kTc \qquad (7.1.9)$$

which is the same as (7.1.2). Note that (7.1.1) is a special case that holds when $c = 0$.

What happens to (7.1.2) when sugar is present on both sides of the membrane? The reader can probably guess that the flow of water is then given by

$$(P_1 - P_2) - kT(c_1 - c_2) = R\,Q \qquad (7.1.10)$$

where c_1 and c_2 are the two concentrations {see Ex. 7.2}. Thus, the concentration *difference* between the two solutions determines their *relative osmotic pressure*.

Finally, what happens when a mixture of solutes is present? It should be clear from the foregoing derivation that the crucial determinant of osmotic pressure is the *number* of independently moving solute particles per unit volume. Thus, in a mixture of solutes, the *partial osmotic pressures* add up, just as the partial pressures add up to determine the total pressure of a mixture of gases. An important example of this is the case of ionic solutions. If $NaCl$ is dissolved in water, the Na^+ and Cl^- ions move independently, and the osmotic pressure of the solution is

$$kT[Na^+] + kT\,[Cl^-]$$

where $[\,]$ denotes concentration.

7.2   A Simple Model of Cell Volume Control

In this section, we describe a simplified model of the mechanism that animal cells use to achieve osmotic balance and control their volume. The simplification is that we ignore all electrical effects. This will be remedied in later sections.

Consider the cell shown in Figure 7.2. In its interior there are some molecules that cannot get through the cell membrane. The number of these molecules is designated by X, so their concentration is X/V where V is the volume of the

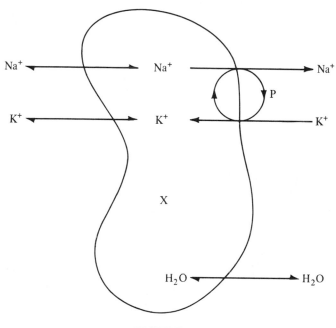

FIGURE 7.2.

cell. The cell also contains Na^+ and K^+ ions. These ions can diffuse through the cell membrane, which is also permeable to water.

In addition, the cell membrane is equipped with a "pump" that pumps internal Na^+ ions out of the cell in exchange for external K^+ ions. This active process is needed to maintain the cell volume constant, as we shall see.

We make the assumption that the pressure inside the cell equals the pressure outside it. That is, we assume that the cell membrane cannot withstand any mechanical pressure difference. In this respect, the cell membrane differs from the rigid membrane considered earlier.

The equations for the net flux of Na^+, K^+, and H_2O in the outward direction are:

$$f_{Na} = \alpha_{Na}([Na^+]_i - [Na^+]_o) + p \qquad (7.2.1)$$

$$f_K = \alpha_K([K^+]_i - [K^+]_o) - p \qquad (7.2.2)$$

$$R_{(H_2O)}Q = -kT([Na^+]_i + [K^+]_i + (X/V) - [Na^+]_o - [K^+]_o). \qquad (7.2.3)$$

In these equations f stands for flux (ions per unit time), and p is the pump rate. The quantities α_{Na} and α_K are the (passive) permeabilities of the cell to Na^+ and K^+, and $R_{(H_2O)}$ is the resistance of the cell membrane to the flow of water. The subscripts i and o designate the inside and the outside of the cell, respectively. Equation (7.2.3) is the osmotic pressure law derived in the previous section, except that here we have $P_i = P_o$, as discussed above.

Now suppose that the cell is in a *steady state*, which means that the net flux of all quantities is zero. Then (7.2.1) through (7.2.3) become

$$[Na^+]_i - [Na^+]_o = -p/\alpha_{Na} \tag{7.2.4}$$

$$[K^+]_i - [K^+]_o = +p/\alpha_K \tag{7.2.5}$$

$$[Na^+]_i + [K^+]_i + (X/V) = [Na^+]_o + [K^+]_o. \tag{7.2.6}$$

Equations (7.2.4) and (7.2.5) give the concentration differences produced by the pump, whereas (7.2.6) simply asserts that the total concentration of solute must be the same inside and outside the cell—otherwise, water would flow. Substituting (7.2.4) and (7.2.5) in (7.2.6), we get

$$\begin{aligned} X/V &= p((1/\alpha_{Na}) - (1/\alpha_K)) \\ &= p(\alpha_K - \alpha_{Na})/(\alpha_K \alpha_{Na}). \end{aligned} \tag{7.2.7}$$

That is,

$$V = (X/p)(\alpha_K \alpha_{Na})/(\alpha_K - \alpha_{Na}). \tag{7.2.8}$$

This result has some interesting implications. First, we get a finite positive[1] cell volume V only if $\alpha_K > \alpha_{Na}$. That is, the cell membrane has to be more permeable to K^+ than to Na^+. This asymmetry is necessary because the pump pushes Na^+ *out* and K^+ *in*. Diffusion through the membrane partially offsets the work of the pump. Therefore, when $\alpha_K > \alpha_{Na}$, the net effect of the pump is to reduce the concentration of ions in the cell. This offsets the molecules that are trapped in the cell and makes it possible for the cell to achieve osmotic balance and a steady state.

The second interesting point is the dependence of V on p. Equation (7.2.8) shows that the cell volume is inversely proportional to the pump rate. As $p \to 0, V \to \infty$. This shows the necessity of the pump for holding the cell volume down. Dead cells swell.

Finally, we note that V is proportional to X. Thus, the volume of our model cell is automatically adjusted to the number of protein and other macromolecules that are trapped within the cell's membrane. As the cell produces more molecules, say through growth, its volume automatically increases proportionally.

7.3 The Movement of Ions across Cell Membranes

A battery is shown in Figure 7.3 to be driving an ionic current across a membrane. The purpose of the battery is to specify the voltage difference

---

[1]The negative value of V that is obtained when $\alpha_K < \alpha_{Na}$ has no physical significance; it merely tells us that there is no steady state volume in this situation. If we studied the time-dependent equations for the case $\alpha_K < \alpha_{Na}$, we would find that V increases indefinitely. In practice, the cell would swell until it burst.

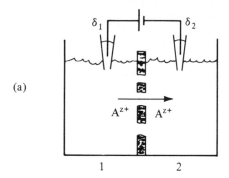

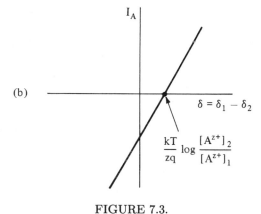

FIGURE 7.3.

across the membrane (also known as the membrane potential) so that we can study the relationship between the membrane potential and the ionic current. Later we shall see how the membrane potential is determined in the physiological situation, where there is, of course, no battery applied to the system from the outside as in Figure 7.3. The ionic current in Fig. 7.3 is carried by a particular ionic species designated by A^{z+}. This notation means that each ion carries z elementary (positive) charges. That is, its charge is zq, where q is the magnitude of the charge on an electron. We are interested here in Na^+ and K^+, for which $z = +1$, and in Cl^-, for which $z = -1$.

The battery establishes a potential difference

$$\delta = \delta_1 - \delta_2$$

and we want to derive the relationship between this potential difference and the current I_A flowing through the membrane.

The relationship shown in Figure 7.3B can be derived from energetic arguments similar to the ones used in Section 3.1. The assumptions that we need are:

1. The work *performed* by the battery per unit time is

$$dW_{battery}/dt = I_A(\delta_1 - \delta_2) = I_A\,\delta. \tag{7.3.1}$$

This follows from the definitions of current and potential since current is charge per unit time and potential (voltage) is work per unit charge.

2. The rate at which work is *required* to drive current through the membrane is

$$dW_{membrane}/dt = R_A I_A^2. \tag{7.3.2}$$

The reader should be warned that this assumption is only correct in particularly simple situations. The actual form of $dW_{membrane}/dt$ depends on the details of the mechanism that transports ions across the membrane. We make the assumption (7.3.2) because it leads to the simplest possible current–voltage relation (as shown in Figure 7.3B) and because this simple relationship is actually observed in some biologically important membranes, such as the squid axons in which the fundamental properties of nerve membranes were discovered.

3. The rate at which work is *required* to change the concentration of the ions from $[A^{z+}]_1$ to $[A^{z+}]_2$ as the ions are driven across the membrane is the same as if the ions were the molecules of an ideal gas. This amount of work is $kT \log([A^{z+}]_2/[A^{z+}]_1)$ per ion transported across the membrane. Since the number of ions transported across the membrane per unit time is $I_A/(zq)$, we have

$$dW_{concentration}/dt = I_A(kT/zq) \log([A^{z+}]_2/[A^{z+}]_1). \tag{7.3.3}$$

By the conversation of energy law, we have that

$$dW_{battery}/dt = dW_{membrane}/dt + dW_{concentration}/dt. \tag{7.3.4}$$

Substituting into this and dividing by IA, we obtain

$$\delta = R_A I_A + (kT/zq) \log([A^{z+}]_2/[A^{z+}]_1). \tag{7.3.5}$$

Dividing by R_A and rearranging terms gives

$$I_A = g_A(\delta - (kT/zq) \log([A^{z+}]_2/[A^{z+}]_1)) \tag{7.3.6}$$

where $g_A = 1/R_A$ is called the *membrane conductance*. This is the current–voltage relationship plotted in Figure 7.3B. The quantity

$$E_A = (kT/zq) \log([A^{z+}]_2/[A^{z+}]_1) \tag{7.3.7}$$

is called the *equilibrium potential* of the ion in question. When $\delta = E_A$, the current is zero. It is worth mentioning here that this expression for the equilibrium potential holds much more generally than the linear current–voltage relation derived here. If assumption (2) were changed, then the current–voltage relation would become nonlinear, but it would still have the same equilibrium potential.

Finally, we apply the results of this section to a situation where several ions are present simultaneously. In that case, we assume that the different ions cross the membrane through different channels; this has been demonstrated experimentally in many cases. Each ion has its own equilibrium potential determined by its concentration ratio, but all of the ions feel the same membrane potential δ. The total current is simply the sum of the individual ionic currents, and each ionic current is given by an expression similar to (7.3.6).

7.4   Control of Cell Volume: The Interaction of Electrical and Osmotic Effects

We now consider the model cell of Figure 7.4, which is an extension of the model that we considered in Section 7.2. Because we now include electrical effects, it is necessary to take into account the Cl^- ions, even though these are not actively transported across the membrane. Also, we now assume that each of the x molecules that are trapped inside the cell carries z negative charges. We therefore designate these molecules by the chemical symbol X^{z-}.

It turns out that the electrical effect of these trapped charges produces an indirect osmotic effect because of the positive ions that are needed to balance the trapped negative charge. This indirect effect is much more important than the direct osmotic effect of X^{z-} when z is large.

We begin by stating the equations of the model cell. Then we discuss the various assumptions contained in these equations. First, we have expressions for the three ionic currents (positive is outward)

$$I_{Na} = g_{Na}(\delta - (kT/q)\log([Na^+]_o/[Na^+]_i)) + pq \qquad (7.4.1)$$

$$I_K = g_K(\delta - (kT/q)\log([K^+]_o/[K^+]_i)) - pq \qquad (7.4.2)$$

$$I_{Cl} = g_{Cl}(\delta + (kT/q)\log([Cl^-]_o/[Cl^-]_i)). \qquad (7.4.3)$$

Next, we have an equation for the membrane potential $\delta = \delta_i - \delta_o$ in terms of the excess charge in the cell:

$$C\,\delta = q(V[Na^+]_i + V[K^+]_i - V[Cl^-]_i - xz) \qquad (7.4.4)$$

where C is the capacitance of the cell membrane, which has the units of charge divided by voltage.

Finally, we have the equation for the osmotic flux of water (again, positive is outward)

$$R_{H_2O}Q = -kT([Na^+]_i + [K^+]_i + [Cl^-]_i + (x/V) - [Na^+]_o - [K^+]_o - [Cl^-]_o). \qquad (7.4.5)$$

The first three equations are the current-voltage relations of the previous section with extra terms added for the currents produced by the pump. If

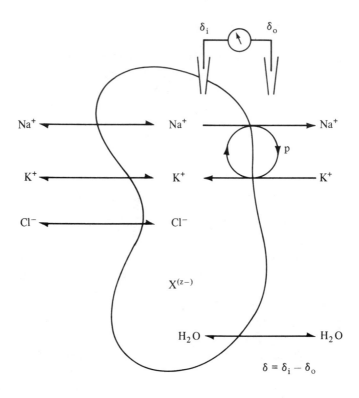

FIGURE 7.4.

p is the pump rate, say in terms of ions exchanged per unit time, then pq is the Na^+ current produced by the pump and $-pq$ is the corresponding K^+ current. Note that the net pump current is zero. We have assumed for simplicity that the pump ratio is 1:1. That is, one Na^+ ion is pumped out of the cell for every K^+ ion that flows inwards via the pump. Equations (7.4.1) and (7.4.2) could easily be changed to accommodate other pump ratios. In the case of a 3:2 pump, for example, Equation (7.4.1) would contain the term $3pq$ and Equation (7.4.2) would contain the term $-2pq$ (instead of pq and $-pq$, respectively).

Since Cl^- is negatively charged, the current I_{Cl} is in the opposite direction to the physical flux of chloride. This explains the change in sign in (7.4.3). It is noteworthy that this change of sign applies only to the equilibrium potential and not to the membrane potential term. This is because the qualitative effect of membrane potential on ionic current is the same for both positive and negative ions. To understand this, recall that a flow of positive charges in one direction and a flow of negative charges in the other are considered as electrical currents flowing in the same direction, that of the positive changes. Thus, a membrane potential which generates positive outward current by pushing positive charges out of the cell also generates positive outward current by pulling negative charges into the cell.

Equation (7.4.4) is based on the assumption that the cell acts like a capacitor so that the membrane potential is proportional to the excess charge. It is important to remark that the excess charge is *very* small compared to the total positive or negative charge. The excellent approximation of setting the excess charge equal to zero is called the condition of *electroneutrality*. It can be obtained mathematically by letting $C \to 0$ in (7.4.4); we shall do this later.

Equation (7.4.5) is the expression for the osmotic flux of water provided we make the assumption, as in Section 7.2, that the membrane cannot withstand any hydrostatic pressure difference so that the internal and external pressures must be equal.

As in Section 7.2, we seek a *steady state* in which the currents I_{Na}, I_K, and I_{Cl} and the water flux Q are all equal to zero. In addition, we make the following simplifications:

1. Let $C = 0$. As remarked above, this yields the condition of electroneutrality, an excellent approximation.

2. Let $xz = N$, so that N is the total number of negative charges that are trapped within the cell. Now consider the limit $z \to \infty$, $x \to 0$ with N fixed. This expresses the fact that the cell contains a relatively small number of large molecules with a large number of negative charges per molecule. The effect of this limit is that the direct osmotic effect of X^{z-} drops out of (7.4.5), but the electrical effect of the negative charge remains in (7.4.4).

When these simplifications have been made, our equations can be rewritten as:

$$0 = g_{Na}(\delta - (kT/q)\log([Na^+]_o/[Na^+]_i)) + pq \qquad (7.4.6)$$

$$0 = g_K(\delta - (kT/q)\log([K^+]_o/[K^+]_i)) - pq \qquad (7.4.7)$$

$$0 = g_{Cl}(\delta + (kT/q)\log([Cl^-]_o/[Cl^-]_i)) \qquad (7.4.8)$$

$$0 = [Na^+]_i + [K^+]_i - [Cl^-]_i - N/V \qquad (7.4.9)$$

$$0 = [Na^+]_i + [K^+]_i + [Cl^-]_i - [Na^+]_o - [K^+]_o - [Cl^-]_o. \qquad (7.4.10)$$

We regard these as five simultaneous equation in the five unknowns $[Na^+]_i$, $[K^+]_i$, $[Cl^-]_i$, δ, and V. The external concentrations are taken to be known. It is important to notice, however, that the given external concentrations must satisfy the equation

$$[Na^+]_o + [K^+]_o = [Cl^-]_o \qquad (7.4.11)$$

so that the external solution is electrically neutral.

To solve this system (7.4.6) through (7.4.10), we proceed as follows. First, we use (7.4.6) through (7.4.8) to express the internal concentrations in terms of the membrane potential δ

$$[Na^+]_i/[Na^+]_o = \exp(-(q\delta/kT) - (pq^2/g_{Na}kT)) \qquad (7.4.12)$$

$$[K^+]_i/[K^+]_o = \exp(-(q\delta/kT) + (pq^2/g_K kT)) \qquad (7.4.13)$$

$$[Cl^-]_i/[Cl^-]_o = \exp(q\delta/kT). \qquad (7.4.14)$$

To simplify the notation, let

$$\gamma = \exp(q\delta/kT) \qquad (7.4.15)$$

$$\beta_{Na} = \exp(-pq^2/g_{Na}kT) \qquad (7.4.16)$$

$$\beta_K = \exp(pq^2/g_K kT) \qquad (7.4.17)$$

so that

$$[Na^+]_i = \gamma^{-1}\beta_{Na}[Na^+]_o \qquad (7.4.18)$$

$$[K^+]_i = \gamma^{-1}\beta_K[K^+]_o \qquad (7.4.19)$$

$$[Cl^-]_i = \gamma[Cl^-]_o. \qquad (7.4.20)$$

These expressions can be substituted into (7.4.9) and (7.4.10) to obtain a pair of equations for γ and V. Note that γ determines δ. After dividing through these equations by $2[Cl^-]_o$ and using (7.4.11), we get

$$0 = \beta/(2\gamma) - \gamma/2 - b \qquad (7.4.21)$$

$$0 = \beta/(2\gamma) + \gamma/2 - 1 \qquad (7.4.22)$$

where

$$b = N/(2[Cl^-]_o V) \qquad (7.4.23)$$

and

$$\beta = (\beta_{Na}[Na^+]_o + \beta_K[K^+]_o)/([Na^+]_o + [K^+]_o). \qquad (7.4.24)$$

We will use (7.4.21), which is the equation of electroneutrality, to express γ in terms of b. This means that we are finding the potential in terms of the cell volume, which is temporarily regarded as given. Later, we use the equation of osmotic balance (7.4.22) to determine the volume.

Equation (7.4.21) can be written as the quadratic

$$\gamma^2/2 + b\,\gamma - \beta/2 = 0. \qquad (7.4.25)$$

The positive solution of (7.4.25) is

$$\gamma = -b + \sqrt{(b^2 + \beta)}. \qquad (7.4.26)$$

We are forced to take the positive solution here because $\gamma = \exp(q\delta/kT)$, which is positive for all δ. Note that

$$1/\gamma = (b + \sqrt{(b^2 + \beta)})/\beta. \qquad (7.4.27)$$

Finally, we can determine b, and hence the cell volume V by substituting (7.4.26) and (7.4.27) in the equation of osmotic balance (7.4.22). The result is

$$\sqrt{(b^2 + \beta)} = 1 \qquad (7.4.28)$$

$$b = \sqrt{(1 - \beta)} \qquad (7.4.29)$$

$$V = N/[2[Cl^-]_o\sqrt{(1 - \beta)}]. \qquad (7.4.30)$$

Thus, we only get real, finite volumes if $\beta < 1$. When $\beta \geq 1$, there is no steady volume possible and the cell swells until it bursts.

We next investigate the dependence of β upon the pump rate p. We have

$$\beta(p) = ([Na^+]_o \exp(-pq^2/g_{Na}kT)+[K^+]_o \exp(pq^2/g_K kT))/([Na^+]_o+[K^+]_o). \qquad (7.4.31)$$

Clearly, $\beta(0) = 1$ and $\beta(p) \to +\infty$ as $p \to +\infty$.
Differentiating this expression, we find that

$$d\beta/dp = a(-[Na^+]_o\beta_{Na}/g_{Na} + [K^+]_o\beta_K/g_K) \qquad (7.4.32)$$

so

$$(d\beta/dp)(0) = a(-[Na^+]_o/g_{Na} + [K^+]_o/g_K) \qquad (7.4.33)$$

where a is independent of p. We now impose the condition

$$[Na^+]_o/g_{Na} > [K^+]_o/g_K \qquad (7.4.34)$$

so that $d\beta/dp < 0$ at $p = 0$. With this inequality satisfied, there is a range of pump rates that lead to finite volume, steady state solutions, since $\beta(p) < 1$

for small enough values of p. If (7.4.34) is not satisfied, it is easy to see that $\beta > 1$ for all $p > 0$, and no such solutions exist.

When (7.4.34) holds, it is interesting to note that β has a minimum at a value of p found by setting $d\beta/dp = 0$. The result is

$$p_{opt} = (kT/q^2)(g_{Na}g_K/(g_{Na} + g_K)) \log([Na^+]_o g_K/g_{Na}[K^+]_o). \qquad (7.4.35)$$

From (7.4.30), we see that this is also the value of p that minimizes the cell volume, V. It seems reasonable to speculate that real cells operate their pumps at a rate that is near p_{opt} because at this pump rate, the cell volume is insensitive to small changes in the pump rate. The quantitative relationship between cell volume and pump rate is further investigated in Exercise 7.5.

At a fixed pump rate, we can see from (7.4.30) and (7.4.31) that the cell volume depends on the number of trapped negative charges and also on the ionic concentrations in the external medium. During cell growth, as more macromolecules carrying trapped negative charges are produced, the cell volume increases proportionally. The dependence of cell volume on external ionic concentrations can be described as follows: First, note that β can be rewritten in terms of the ratio $[Na^+]_o/[K^+]_o$. When this ratio is fixed, the cell volume is inversely proportional to the total external ion concentration $2[Cl^-]_o = [Cl^-]_o + [Na^+]_o + [K^+]_o$. Thus, cells swell in a more dilute external environment.

Moreover, if the ratio $[Na^+]_o/[K^+]_o$ is reduced, then β increases and the cell volume also increases. In fact, as we have remarked above, if the ratio $[Na^+]_o/[K^+]_o$ is so low that (7.4.34) is violated, then the cell volume becomes infinite; i.e., the cell bursts. Thus, the cell volume is sensitive both to the total external ion concentration and also to the composition of the external medium.

Finally, with the cell volume known, we can determine the steady state, or resting, membrane potential δ. To do this, we substitute (7.4.29) in (7.4.26). The result is

$$\gamma = -\sqrt{(1 - \beta)} + 1 \qquad (7.4.36)$$

so that

$$\delta = (kT/q) \log \gamma = (kT/q) \log(1 - \sqrt{(1 - \beta)}). \qquad (7.4.37)$$

Since $\gamma < 1, \delta < 0$. Thus, the negative membrane potential of animal cells is a by-product of the mechanism that regulates cell volume. In the next section, we shall see how the membrane potential can be transiently modified by changes in the passive conductances g_{Na} and g_K. This is the basis of the signaling mechanism that is used for communication by nerve and muscle cells.

7.5   Transient Changes in Membrane Potential: A Signaling Mechanism in Nerve and Muscle

The basic mechanism for control of cell volume that we have outlined above operates in all animal cells. But, nerve cells and muscle cells also have the ability to make brief changes in the membrane potential by adjusting the conductances g_K and g_{Na}. These changes lead to departures from the steady state so that I_{Na}, I_K and I_{Cl} are not equal to zero. Nevertheless, if we make the approximation $C = 0$, which leads to electroneutrality, then we must have

$$I_{Na} + I_K + I_{Cl} = 0 \qquad (7.5.1)$$

{see Ex. 7.7}.

Substituting (7.4.1) through (7.4.3) into this equation, we find that Na^+ and K^+ pump currents cancel and that

$$\delta = (g_{Na}E_{Na} + g_K E_K + g_{Cl}E_{Cl})/(g_{Na} + g_K + g_{Cl}) \qquad (7.5.2)$$

where

$$E_{Na} = (kT/q)\log([Na^+]_o/[Na^+]_i) \qquad (7.5.3)$$

$$E_K = (kT/q)\log([K^+]_o/[K^+]_i) \qquad (7.5.4)$$

$$E_{Cl} = (kT/-q)\log([Cl^-]_o/[Cl^-]_i). \qquad (7.5.5)$$

Thus, the membrane potential is a weighted average of the equilibrium potentials of the various ions. The weights are the conductances g_{Na}, g_K, and g_{Cl}. By varying the conductances, the membrane potential can be shifted between $E_K = -100 \ mV$ and $E_{Na} = +55 \ mV$. This is the physical mechanism that is used to generate signals that propagate along the membranes of nerve cells and muscle cells {see Ex. 7.6}.

7.6 Annotated References

This Chapter introduces the subject of osmotic pressure and osmotic flow across membranes. For a comprehensive treatment of this subject, see the following monograph:

Finkelstein, A.: *Water Movement Through Lipid Bilayers, Pores, and Plasma Membranes: Theory and Reality* (Distinguished Lecture Series of the Society of General Physiologists, Volume 4), Wiley, New York, 1987.

The type of model used here for the control of cell volume was pioneered by Tosteson and Hoffman:

Tosteson, D.C. and Hoffman, J.F.: Regulation of cell volume by active cation transport in high and low potassium sheep red cells. *Journal of General Physiology* **44**: 169–194, 1960.

Tosteson, D.C.: Regulation of cell volume by sodium and potassium transport. In: *The Cellular Functions of Membrane Transport* (Hoffman, J.F., ed.) Society of General Physiologists Symposium #10, Prentice Hall, New York, NY, 1964.

This Chapter provides an introduction to the membrane physiology that is needed to understand the electrical signalling mechanisms of nerve and muscle. This is a vast subject in which the most important single work is the following:

Hodgkin, A.L. and Huxley, A.F: A quantitative description of membrane current and its application to conduction and excitation in nerve. *Journal of Physiology* **117**, 500–544, 1952.

Exercises

7.1. WORK

In mechanics, work = force × distance. If a force f is applied through a distance ds, the amount of work performed is $dW = f\, ds$.

Consider a piston with cross-sectional area A that applies a pressure (force/area) P to a fluid as it moves through a distance dx. Show that the work done is $dW = P\, dV$, where dV is the volume displaced by the piston.

7.2. EQUATION FOR FLOW WHEN THERE IS SOLUTE ON BOTH SIDES
OF THE MEMBRANE

Derive Equation (7.1.10).

7.3. OSMOTIC PRESSURE

Suppose that 180 g of sugar are dissolved in enough water to make up 10^3 cm^3 of sugar solution. Calculate the osmotic pressure of this solution at $T = 300°K$, given the following data:

1. the weight of a sugar molecule is 3.0×10^{-22} g

2. Boltzmann's constant is $k = 1.4 \times 10^{-16}$ dyne-cm/°K.

How high could this amount of pressure raise a column of water whose cross-sectional area is 1 cm^2? To figure this out, you need to know that the force of gravity on 1 cm^3 of water is 980 dynes. What if the cross-sectional area of the water column is 10^6 cm^2?

7.4. WORK OF COMPRESSION

Suppose that n molecules of an ideal gas are compressed by a piston from volume V_1, where the concentration is $c_1 = n/V_1$, to a volume V_2 where the concentration is $c_2 = n/V_2$. While the compression is occurring, the temperature is held constant at the value T. Show that the work performed by the piston is $nkT \log(c_2/c_1)$. (Hint: Use $dW = -P\, dV$ and $P = nkT/V$. Integrate from V_1 to V_2, and express the result in terms of concentration.)

7.5. THE EFFECT OF PUMP RATE ON CELL VOLUME AND
MEMBRANE POTENTIAL

In this exercise, use the data:

$$g_{Na} = 3.3\mu\text{mho}/cm^2$$

$$
\begin{aligned}
g_K &= 240 \mu\text{mho/cm}^2 \\
[Na^+]_o &= 145 \ \mu M/\text{cm}^3 \\
[K^+]_o &= 4 \ \mu M/\text{cm}^3 \\
q &= 1.6 \times 10^{-19} \ \text{coulombs} \\
kT/q &= 25 \times 10^{-3} \ \text{volts}
\end{aligned}
$$

where $\mu mho = 10^{-6}$ (coulomb/sec)/volt, a mho is the basic unit of conductance (the reciprocal of resistance, measured in ohms), the coulomb is a standard unit of charge, and $1\mu M = 10^{-6} \times (6 \times 10^{23})$ ions.

1. Check that (7.4.34) is satisfied.

2. Plot β, V, and δ against p over the range of p values for which $\beta < 1$. Plot V in units of $N/2[Cl^-]_o$ and δ in units of kT/q.

3. Evaluate p_{opt} from Equation (7.4.35) and check that V and δ have minima at $p = p_{opt}$.

4. Assuming that $p = p_{opt}$, evaluate $[Na^+]_i$, $[K^+]_i$, and $[Cl^-]_i$. Also, evaluate δ.

5. Still assuming that $p = p_{opt}$, evaluate E_{Na}, E_K, and E_{Cl} in equations (7.5.3) through (7.5.5). Note that $E_{Cl} = \delta$. Why is this? Similarly, this problem is solved without specifying a value for g_{Cl}. How is this possible?

7.6. THE NERVE IMPULSE

Using Equation (7.5.2) and the values of E_{Na}, E_K, and E_{Cl} calculated above, evaluate δ under the following conditions (i.e., complete the following table):

	I	II	III	
t	0	0.25	1.0	ms (10^{-3} s)
g_{Na}	3.3	30,000	3.3	μ mho/cm^2
g_K	240	3000	3000	μ mho/cm^2
g_{Cl}	300	300	300	μ mho/cm^2
δ	—	—	—	

Sketch the graph of the behavior of δ as a function of time if the conductances go through a sequence of values $I \to II \to III \to I$. The return to state I takes about 10 ms. The signal that you have constructed is a nerve impulse.

7.7 Zero Capacitance

Assuming that $C = 0$, derive (7.5.1). (Hint: Since we are not in the steady state, the internal concentrations change with time.) Thus, we have the equations

$$d(V[Na^+]_i)/dt \;=\; I_{Na}/q$$
$$d(V[K^+]_i)/dt \;=\; I_K/q$$
$$d(V[Cl^-]_i)/dt \;=\; I_{Cl}/(-q).$$

Add these equations and use (7.4.4) with $C = 0$.

8

The Renal Countercurrent Mechanism

The function of the kidney is to regulate the composition of the blood *plasma*. The plasma is the part of the blood that remains when the cells have been removed. We shall consider only the regulation of the Na^+ content of the blood plasma, but the reader should keep in mind that the kidney is actually regulating the concentrations of many other substances at the same time.

In an organism with a variable diet, the kidney can only achieve a constant Na^+ concentration in blood plasma if it is able to produce urine in which Na^+ is either more or less concentrated than in plasma according to the needs of the moment. If a salty meal has just been consumed, for example, the kidney needs to excrete urine in which the Na^+ concentration is greater than that of the blood plasma. If, on the other hand, a large quantity of fresh water has just been consumed, then the kidney needs to excrete urine in which the salt concentration is less than the plasma's.

In this chapter, we describe the simplest mathematical theory that can account for this dual capability in a reasonably realistic way.

8.1   The Nephron

The basic unit of the renal function is the *nephron*, shown in Figure 8.1. The kidney is made up of about 10^6 nephrons that are connected in parallel with each other, both with respect to their blood supply and with respect to the production of urine. We will describe the function of the nephron in terms of its different parts.

The transformation from blood plasma to urine begins at the *glomerulus* (G). Blood enters the glomerulus through an *afferent arteriole* (AA) that breaks up into a network of glomerular capillaries. The walls of these capillaries are permeable to water and small molecules. These substances are said to be *filtered* out of the capillaries.

The protein molecules in blood plasma are too large to be filtered, and their osmotic pressure opposes the process of filtration. Moreover, the small ions that are needed to balance the fixed charges on the proteins also contribute to the effective osmotic pressure of the proteins. (Protein molecules are often charged because several of the amino acids from which proteins are assembled contain chemical groups on their side chains that are ionized at physiological pH values.) This combined osmotic effect opposing the process of filtration is

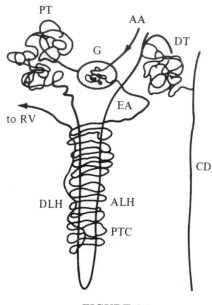

FIGURE 8.1.

called *oncotic pressure*. It must be overcome by the blood pressure for filtration to proceed.

When fluid leaves the glomerulus, it enters the *proximal convoluted tubule* (PT). The proximal tubular fluid has essentially the composition of blood plasma without the proteins. In the proximal tubule, Na^+ is actively reabsorbed from the tubular fluid, but the walls are permeable to water, which follows the Na^+ for osmotic reasons. Thus, the Na+ concentration in the proximal tubule remains that of blood plasma, but the volume of fluid flowing out the end of the proximal tubule per unit time is less than the volume of fluid filtered.

Changes in Na^+ concentration begin in the *loop of Henle*. The active part of the loop, i.e., the place where metabolic energy is used, is the *ascending limb* (ALH) where Na^+ is pumped out of the tubules against a concentration difference into the interstitial fluid. The ascending limb is impermeable to water, so water is trapped in the tubule and cannot follow the Na^+. The consequences of this Na^+ flux out of the ascending limb are not obvious and they can best be predicted with the help of a mathematical model: The result of the Na^+ flux is that the Na^+ concentration in the interstitial fluid (outside the tubules) increases dramatically with depth, so that the concentration is highest at the bend of Henle's loop where the descending limb joins the ascending limb.

Thus, fluid in the *descending limb* of Henle's loop (DLH) flows through a medium in which the Na^+ concentration increases progressively. The walls of the descending limb are permeable to Na^+ and water, so Na^+ flows in and water flows out, concentrating the tubular fluid as it descends. In fact, the walls of the descending tubule are so permeable that the internal and external Na^+ concentrations are nearly equal.

Overall, the operation of Henle's loop results in the removal of Na^+ and water from the tubular fluid. The excess Na^+ and water are picked up by the *peritubular capillaries* (PTC) and returned to the *renal vein* (RV). These capillaries are remarkable in that they are connected in series with the glomerular capillaries via the *efferent arteriole* (EA), a structure that is peculiar to the kidney. Because the filtration process at the glomerulus holds back the plasma proteins, blood entering the peritubular capillaries has a higher concentration of plasma proteins than usual. Presumably, the resulting oncotic pressure helps draw the excess water and Na^+ into the peritubular capillaries.

Because of the operation of Henle's loop, the fluid outside the tubules of the loop is more concentrated than the blood plasma, while the tubular fluid leaving the loop is more dilute. This is the basis of the kidney's dual capability to excrete urine that is either more concentrated or more dilute than blood plasma.

The choice between these two modes of operation is made by the pituitary gland, which secretes *antidiuretic hormone* (ADH). When ADH is absent, the walls of the *distal convoluted tubule* (DT) and of the *collecting duct* (CD) are impermeable to water, so the volume of urine is essentially that of the fluid that leaves the top of the ascending limb of Henle's loop. In this situation, which is sometimes called a state of *diuresis*, the kidney excretes a large volume of dilute urine. In some individuals, production of ADH is reduced or absent, and a state of diuresis persists. This is the disease *diabetes insipidus*.

When ADH is present, however, the walls of the distal convoluted tubule and collecting ducts become permeable to water. In the distal convoluted tubule enough water is withdrawn (osmotically) to bring the concentration of solutes back to the level of the blood plasma. Then, as the tubular fluid descends in the collecting duct, enough water is withdrawn to equilibrate with the local interstitial concentration at each level. Thus, the urine ends up with a solute concentration equal to that at the bottom of Henle's loop, a concentration much higher than that of the blood plasma. Moreover, because this high concentration is achieved by withdrawal of water, the volume of urine excreted per unit time is much lower than before. This state, achieved by the action of ADH on the distal nephron, is called a state of *antidiuresis*.

Note that the operation of the concentrating engine of Henle's loop is the same whether the kidney is concentrating the urine or diluting it.

In the foregoing description, we omitted any specific discussion of Na^+ flux in the *distal* nephron. In fact, Na^+ is actively reabsorbed in the distal nephron in exchange for other solutes, and this exchange is important in the control of total body Na^+ content. The (adrenocortical) hormonal mechanisms that regulate this exchange are outside the scope of this chapter, however. We model the distal nephron as though its walls are impermeable to Na^+ ions.

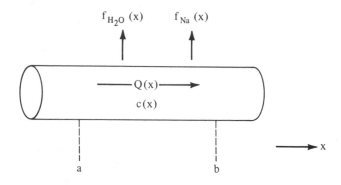

FIGURE 8.2.

8.2   Differential Equations of Na^+ and H_2O Transport along the Renal Tubules

First, consider water transport in the tubule shown in Figure 8.2. The volume rate of flow along the tubule past x is designated by $Q(x)$. We assume that the flow is *steady*, which means that it is independent of time. The volume rate of flow through the walls per unit length near x is designated by $f_{H_2O}(x)$. Our sign convention is that positive Q stands for flow in the direction of increasing x and that positive f stands for outward flux through walls.

To get a differential equation that relates Q and f, consider the segment of tubule that lies between $x = a$ and $x = b$. Since the flow is steady, the volume of this segment cannot change, and the flow into the segment must equal the sum of the flow out of the segment and the flux of water out through the walls of the tube between $x = a$ and $x = b$. In symbols, we have:

$$Q(a) = Q(b) + \int_a^b f_{H_2O}(x)\, dx. \qquad (8.2.1)$$

Thinking of b as a variable and differentiating with respect to b (with a fixed), we get

$$0 = (dQ/dx)(b) + f_{H_2O}(b). \qquad (8.2.2)$$

Since b is arbitrary, this can be written as

$$0 = dQ/dx + f_{H_2O}(x) \qquad (8.2.3)$$

which is the required relationship. If the walls are impermeable to water, $f_{H_2O} = 0$ and (8.2.3) says that $Q = $ constant.

Next, consider Na^+ transport in the same tubule. Let Na^+ concentration in the tubule be $c(x)$. Then the amount of Na^+ per unit time transported along the tubule by the flow past the point x is $Q(x)c(x)$. Let the amount

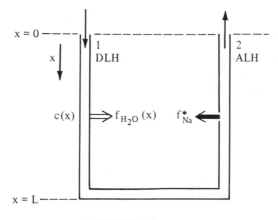

FIGURE 8.3.

of Na^+ per unit time per unit length transported outward through the walls near x be $f_{Na}(x)$. Then an argument identical to the one given above shows that

$$0 = (d/dx)(cQ) + f_{Na}(x). \tag{8.2.4}$$

In a tubule whose walls are impermeable to Na^+, $f_{Na} = 0$, and (8.2.4) says that $cQ -$ constant.

Equations (8.2.3) and (8.2.4) are general, and they apply to all of the tubules of the kidney. The tubules differ according to the properties of their walls as reflected in the fluxes f_{H_2O} and f_{Na}.

8.3   The Loop of Henle

We shall construct a model of the nephron beginning with the most interesting part of the system, the loop of Henle (see Figure 8.3). The descending limb of the loop is designated tube 1 and the ascending limb tube 2. The Na^+ concentrations and water flows in the tubules are written $c_i(x)$ and $Q_i(x)$, respectively, where $i = 1, 2$. The external Na^+ concentration is denoted by $c(x)$. By our sign conventions, the flow is positive in the descending limb and negative in the ascending limb, since x increases downward.

The physiological assumptions of our model of Henle's loop are:

1. We assume that the walls of the descending limb are permeable to water but not to Na^+. This is a simplification: The walls are also permeable to Na^+, but this is not an essential feature of the operation of Henle's loop, and we leave it out. Moreover, we assume that the water permeablility is so large that the water flux makes the internal and external Na^+ concentrations equal. This gives the equations

$$0 = dQ_1/dx + f_{H_2O}^{(1)}(x) \tag{8.3.1}$$

$$0 = (d/dx)(Q_1 c_1) \tag{8.3.2}$$

$$c_1(x) = c(x). \tag{8.3.3}$$

2. We assume that Na^+ is pumped out of the ascending limb at a fixed rate f_{Na}^* per unit length. We also assume that the ascending limb is impermeable to water. This gives

$$0 = dQ_2/dx \tag{8.3.4}$$

$$0 = (d/dx)(Q_2 c_2) + f_{Na}^*. \tag{8.3.5}$$

3. At the turn of Henle's loop ($x = L$) we assume that all of the salt and water leaving the descending limb enter the ascending limb. This gives the boundary conditions

$$c_1(L) = c_2(L) \tag{8.3.6}$$

$$Q_1(L) = -Q_2(L). \tag{8.3.7}$$

4. Finally, we need an assumption about the *peritubular capillaries*, which pick up the Na^+ that is actively pumped out of the ascending limb and the water that passively flows out of the descending limb. First, we assume that the capillaries pick up this Na^+ and water locally. That is, we do not allow for any longitudinal flow outside of the tubules and capillaries. Since we are considering a steady state model, it follows that the peritubular capillaries pick up water at the rate $f_{H_2O}^{(1)}(x)$ and Na^+ at the rate f_{Na}^* per unit length. The detailed mechanism of water and Na^+ transport across the capillary walls can give us additional equations, however. Here, we assume that the interstitial fluid is picked up by a process of filtration analogous to the process that occurs in the glomerular capillaries but running here in the opposite direction. The driving force for this reverse filtration is provided by the oncotic pressure of the plasma proteins. As remarked above, these proteins are present in higher concentrations in the peritubular capillaries than in the rest of the circulation because they were held back by the filtration process at the glomerulus. In reverse filtration at the peritubular capillaries, we assume that the Na^+ is carried passively by the water at its local tissue concentration. This implies a relationship between the flux of Na^+ and the flow of water:

$$f_{Na}^* = c(x) f_{H_2O}^{(1)}(x). \tag{8.3.8}$$

It is a remarkable feature of the model that we do not need to specify any more details about the peritubular capillaries than the considerations that lead to (8.3.8). We now have enough equations to determine $c(x)$ without reference to any further properties of the peritubular capillaries. This would not have been true if different assumptions about Na^+ and water transport across the capillary walls had been made.

We begin the study of Henle's loop by deriving a differential equation for the interstitial concentration $c(x)$. Note that (8.3.1) and (8.3.2) can be rewritten using (8.3.3) and (8.3.8) as follows:

$$0 = (dQ_1/dx) + f_{Na}^*/c(x) \tag{8.3.9}$$

$$0 = (d/dx)(Q_1 c). \tag{8.3.10}$$

Now, (8.3.10) implies that $Q_1 c = $ constant. We use this to get an expression for $Q_1(x)$ in terms of $c(x)$:

$$Q_1(x) = Q_1(0)c(0)/c(x). \tag{8.3.11}$$

Note that $c(0)$ is the Na^+ concentration $c(x)$ in the fluid entering the loop of Henle from the proximal tubule. This is the same as the Na^+ concentration in blood plasma, and we can therefore regard $c(0)$ as given. Similarly, $Q_1(0)$ is the volume rate of flow entering the loop. This flow is *less* than the filtration rate by the total amount of fluid reabsorbed in the proximal tubule per unit time. We will see later how $Q_1(0)$ is determined.

Another consequence of (8.3.10) is that

$$c(dQ_1/dx) = -Q_1 dc/dx = -Q_1(0)c(0)(dc/dx)/c(x). \tag{8.3.12}$$

It follows that (8.3.9) can be rewritten in the form

$$dc/dx = f_{Na}^* c/(Q_1(0)c(0)) \tag{8.3.13}$$

which implies that

$$c(x) = c(0)\exp(f_{Na}^* x/(Q_1(0)c(0))) \tag{8.3.14}$$

and, in particular that

$$c(L) = c(0)\exp(f_{Na}^* L/(Q_1(0)c(0))). \tag{8.3.15}$$

Note that $f_{Na}^* L$ is the total rate at which Na^+ is actively pumped out through the walls of the ascending limb of Henle's loop, while $Q_1(0)c(0)$ is the rate at which Na^+ enters the loop from the proximal tubule. Thus, the ratio of these fluxes

$$\alpha = f_{Na}^* L/(Q_1(0)c(0)) < 1 \tag{8.3.16}$$

determines the maximum concentrating ability of the model nephron for Na+ through the equation

$$c(L) = c(0)\exp(\alpha). \tag{8.3.17}$$

We are now ready to consider the ascending limb of Henle's loop. Since this tubule is impermeable to water (equation 8.3.4) we have

$$\begin{aligned} Q_2(x) &= Q_2(L) = -Q_1(L) \\ &= -Q_1(0)c(0)/c(L) \\ &= -Q_1(0)\exp(-\alpha). \end{aligned} \tag{8.3.18}$$

Since Q_2 is constant, Equation (8.3.5) reduces to

$$dc/dx = f_{Na}^*/(-Q_2) = f_{Na}^* \exp(\alpha)/Q_1(0). \tag{8.3.19}$$

It follows that

$$c_2(x) = c_2(L) + (x - L)f_{Na}^* \exp(\alpha)/Q_1(0). \tag{8.3.20}$$

But, $c_2(L) = c(L) = c(0)\exp(\alpha)$. Thus,

$$c_2(x) = c(0)\exp(\alpha) + (x - L)f_{Na}^* \exp(\alpha)/Q_1(0). \tag{8.3.21}$$

In particular,

$$\begin{aligned}
c_2(0) &= c(0)\exp(\alpha) + (0 - L)f_{Na}^* \exp(\alpha)/Q_1(0) \\
&= c(0)\exp(\alpha)(1 - \alpha).
\end{aligned} \tag{8.3.22}$$

It is now easy to check {see Exercise 8.2} that $\exp(\alpha)(1 - \alpha) < 1$ when $\alpha \neq 0$. Thus, $c_2(0) < c(0)$ and the fluid leaving the top of the ascending limb is more dilute than blood plasma.

We have succeeded in expressing the outputs of Henle's loop in terms of its inputs. In the next section, we will find a good physiological reason for reversing this procedure. That is, we will find that the nephron actually adjusts $Q_1(0)$ to achieve a specified Na^+ concentration $c_2(0)$ at the top of the ascending limb. Thus, we should regard $c_2(0)$ as being a parameter, and we should express $Q_1(0)$ in terms of it.

8.4 The Juxtaglomerular Apparatus and the Renin-Angiotensin System

Near the top of the ascending limb of Henle's loop there is a specialized cluster of cells called the *juxtaglomerular apparatus*. These cells monitor the tubular fluid and secrete a hormone, *renin*, into the afferent arteriole just before it enters the glomerulus. Renin is converted in the blood to *angiotensin*, a potent vasoconstrictor, i.e., a substance that stimulates the constriction of blood vessels. Although the details are not certain, it is a plausible hypothesis that the cells of the juxtaglomerular apparatus monitor specifically the Na^+ concentration at the top of the ascending limb, and that they secrete enough renin to make the glomerular filtration, and perhaps reabsorption from the proximal tubule, proceed at whatever rate is needed to achieve a target level Na^+ concentration at that site. Evidence that such a feedback mechanism is in operation comes from experiments of Thurau, who was able to shut down flow in the proximal nephron by perfusing the distal nephron with salt solutions of higher than normal concentration.

We will model this feedback mechanism in the simplest possible way: We assume that the inflow $Q_1(0)$ to the loop of Henle takes on whatever value is needed to satisfy the equation

$$c_2(0) = c^* \tag{8.4.1}$$

where $c^* < c(0)$ is the target concentration sought by the juxtaglomerular apparatus. Thus, we do not model the details of the renin-angiotensin system. We simply assume it is working and we study its effects on the performance of the nephron.

Substituting (8.3.22) in (8.4.1), we get

$$a = \exp(\alpha)(1 - \alpha) \tag{8.4.2}$$

where

$$a = c^*/c(0) < 1. \tag{8.4.3}$$

Here a is regarded as known $(0 < a < 1)$, so (8.4.2) is an equation for α and hence for $Q_1(0)$.

The graphical solution of (8.4.2) is discussed in Exercise 8.3 where it is shown that (8.4.2) has a unique positive solution for each a such that $0 < a < 1$ and that the solution satisfies $0 < \alpha < 1$. Armed with this knowledge, we can see directly from (8.4.2) that as $a \to 0$, $\alpha \to 1$. Thus, for small values of a,

$$\alpha \cong 1 \tag{8.4.4}$$

$$1 - \alpha \cong a/\exp(1) = a/e \tag{8.4.5}$$

from the definition of α, (8.3.16), we see that $\alpha \cong 1$ means that the Na^+ flux entering the loop of Henle has been adjusted to the pumping capacity of the ascending limb.

We can now rewrite the results of the previous section with c^* as a parameter under the assumption that a is small. We have

$$Q_1(0) = f_{Na}^* L/c(0) \tag{8.4.6}$$

$$-Q_2 = f_{Na}^* L/(e\, c(0)) \tag{8.4.7}$$

$$c(L) = e\, c(0) \tag{8.4.8}$$

$$c_2(0) = c^*. \tag{8.4.9}$$

These simple results summarize the behavior of the model of Henle's loop as controlled by the juxtaglomerular apparatus. Equation (8.4.6) states that the inflow to Henle's loop is adjusted so that the amount of Na^+ in entering the loop per unit time $(Q_1(0)c(0))$ is equal to the amount that can be pumped out of the ascending limb per unit time $(f_{Na}^* L)$. Equation (8.4.7) states that the flow $(-Q_2)$ in the ascending limb of the loop is smaller by a factor of $e \cong 2.7$ than the flow entering the loop $(Q_1(0))$. The difference of course was reabsorbed from the descending limb and carried away by the peritubular capillaries along with the Na^+ pumped out of the ascending limb. Equation (8.4.8) states that the Na^+ concentration outside the tubules (and also in the descending limb of Henle's loop) increases by a factor of e as we follow the descending limb from its origin (where the Na^+ concentration is $c(0)$, the same as in blood plasma) to its turning point (where the Na^+ concentration is $c(L)$). Finally, Equation (8.4.9) states that the Na^+ concentration in the fluid

TABLE 8.1. Outputs of the Model Nephron

		Diluting Mode (ADH Absent)	Concentrating Mode (ADH Present)
Na^+	concentration in urine	c^*	$e\,c(0)$
Rate	of H_2O excretion	$f_{Na}^*L/(ec(0))$	$f_{Na}^*Lc^*/(ec(0))^2$
Rate	of Na^+ excretion	$f_{Na}^*L\,c^*/(ec(0))$	$f_{Na}^*Lc^*/(ec(0))$

leaving the loop of Henle at the top of the ascending limb has the "target" Na^+ concentration c^*, which was indirectly established by the flow regulation achieved by the juxtaglomerular apparatus. Equations (8.4.6) through (8.4.9) are approximate results that are valid only when $c^* << c(0)$.

8.5   The Distal Tubule and Collecting Duct: Concentrating and Diluting Modes

We now come to the stage in the formation of urine where a decision has to be made whether to excrete a large volume of dilute urine or a small volume of concentrated urine. The hormone that determines which possibility will occur is antidiuretic hormone (ADH). When ADH is absent, we assume that the distal tubule and the collecting ducts are simple conduits, impermeable to both salt and water. In these circumstances, the fluid that leaves the top of the ascending limb becomes urine without further modification. Its properties are summarized in the first column of Table 8.1.

When ADH is present, the situation is more complicated. The effect of ADH is to make the distal tubule and the collecting duct permeable to water. We assume that this permeability is so great that equilibrium is achieved at every stage. In the distal convoluted tubule then, enough water is withdrawn to make the Na^+ concentration equal to that of the blood plasma. Then, in the collecting duct, enough water is withdrawn to equilibrate with $c(x)$ at each x. We make the approximation that this water flux is negligible compared to the flux coming out of the descending limb {see Ex. 8.6}. It follows that the concentration of Na^+ in the urine is $c(L) = e\,c(0)$. To figure out the volume rate of urine production, we first note that since only water is withdrawn, the Na^+ flux at the end of the collecting duct must be the same as that leaving Henle's loop. This Na^+ flux is given by

$$-Q_2c^* = f_{Na}^*Lc^*/(ec(0)).$$
(8.5.1)

Thus, the flow leaving the collecting duct when ADH is present must be

$$Q_3(L) = -Q_2c^*/c(L) = f_{Na}^*Lc^*/(ec(0))^2.$$
(8.5.2)

These results are entered in the second column of Table 8.1.

Comparison of the two modes of operation of the model nephron can be summarized as follows: First, the urine is more dilute than blood plasma when ADH is absent and more concentrated when ADH is present. Second, the volume rate of flow is much smaller when ADH is present by a factor of $c^*/ec(0)$. The rate at which Na^+ is excreted is the same in both cases, however.

Thus, the ADH mechanism cannot be used to regulate the total Na^+ *content* of the body. It can be used to regulate the Na^+ *concentration* of the blood plasma by excreting varying amounts of water in response to fluctuations in the plasma concentration of Na^+.

8.6 Remarks on the Significance of the Juxtaglomerular Apparatus

The filtration rate in the kidney is about 100 times the rate of urine formation. Therefore, 99% of the filtrate must be reabsorbed, and a 1% error in the reabsorption rate results in a 100% error in the rate of urine formation. A nephron in which filtration is maintained, but reabsorption fails completely, excretes about 100 times as much urine as it should. It is inconceivable that such large errors would be tolerated. Clearly, the kidney needs control mechanisms that adjust the input to each nephron according to the capacity of the nephron for reabsorption of Na^+ and water.

We have seen that the juxtaglomerular apparatus can achieve this end by monitoring the Na^+ concentration at the top of the ascending limb of Henle's loop. When this has been done and when the filtration rate has been adjusted accordingly in each nephron, a heterogeneous population of nephrons can function in a coordinated fashion as easily as a homogeneous population. To see this, note that the concentrations in Table 8.1 are independent of the reabsorption capacity $f^*_{Na} L$ while the rates of excretion of both Na^+ and water are proportional to that capacity.

Thus, each nephron contributes what it can to the production of a homogeneous urine. Coordinated performance of this kind would be impossible without the juxtaglomerular apparatus.

8.7   Annotated References

For students who want to learn more about the physiology of the kidney, the following two texts should be useful (the first is elementary and the second is advanced):

Sullivan, L.P., and Grantham, J.J.: *Physiology of the Kidney* (2nd edition). Lea & Febiger, Philadelphia, 1982.

Koushanpour, E. and Kriz, W.: *Renal Physiology: Principles, Strucutre, and Function* (2nd edition). Springer-Verlag, New York, NY, 1986.

The discussion of the juxtaglomerular apparatus in this Chapter is strongly influenced by the work of Thurau:

Thurau, K. and Mason, J.: Intrarenal function of the juxtaglomerular apparatus. In: *Kidney and Urinary Tract Physiology* (Thurau, K., ed.). M.T.P. International Review of Science, Physiology Series 1, Volume 6. University Park Press, Baltimore, MD, 1974, 357–390.

There is a considerable body of mathematical work concerning the kidney. This literature is reviewed in the following papers:

Knepper, M.A., and Rector, F.C., Jr.: Urinary concnetrationa nd dilution. In: *The Kidney* (4th edition) Volume 1, (Brenner, B.M. and Rector, F.C., Jr., eds.) Harcourt Brace Javanovich, Philadelphia, PA, 1991, 445–482.

Roy, D.R., Layton, H.E., and Jamison, R.L.: Countercurrent mechanism and its regulation. In: *The Kidney: Physiology and Pathophysiology* (2nd edition) (Seldin, D.W. and Giebish, G., eds.) Raven Press, New York, NY, in press.

Exercises

8.1. EQUATION OF Na^+ CONSERVATION IN A RENAL TUBE

Derive Equation (8.2.4).

8.2. CALCULATION

Show that $\exp(\alpha)(1 - \alpha) < 1$ for all $\alpha \neq 0$. (Hint: Consider the sign of the derivative of this function of α when $\alpha > 0$ and when $\alpha < 0$.)

8.3. GRAPHICAL SOLUTION OF THE EQUATION FOR α

Consider the equation $a = \exp(\alpha)(1 - \alpha)$ where a is given and $0 < a < 1$. Plot the right-hand side as a function of α over the interval $0 < \alpha < 1$ and indicate how such a plot could be used to find the unique positive value of α that satisfies the equation. For example, calculate α when $= c^*/c(0) = 0.43$.

8.4. QUANTITATIVE STATE OF THE NEPHRON

Assume that

$$
\begin{aligned}
c(0) &= 140 \text{ mEq/liter} \\
c^* &= 60 \text{ mEq/liter} \\
f^*_{Na}L/c(0) &= 0.25/(2.0 \times 10^6) \text{ liters/minute}
\end{aligned}
$$

where $1 \, mEq = 10^{-3} \times 6.0 \times 10^{23}$ ions.

1. Using the approximation that $c^*/c(0) << 1$, calculate $Q_1(0)$, $Q_1(L)$, $Q_3(0)$, $Q_3(L)$ and $c(L)$. Do this calculation for both the concentrating and diluting modes and use your answers in each case to construct a quantitative diagram of the nephron with flows and Na^+ concentrations labeled at appropriate sites.

2. Repeat part 1, but without making the approximation that $c^*/c(0) << 1$. (Hint: Start from the value of α that was determined in Exercise 8.3.)

8.5. THE EFFECT OF A CHANGE IN f^*_{Na}

What happens to the nephron in Exercise 8.4 (in the concentrating mode) if f^*_{Na} is reduced by a factor of 2? Consider two cases:

1. The juxtaglomerular apparatus is working, so $c_2(0) = c^*$, which remains constant, but $Q_1(0)$ changes.

2. The juxtaglomerular apparatus is not working, so $c_2(0)$ is allowed to change, but $Q_1(0)$ remains constant.

Note: Do *not* use the approximation $c^*/c(0) << 1$.

Compare the two cases with regard to water output, Na^+ output, and Na^+ concentration in the urine. What happens in the two cases if $f^*_{Na} = 0$?

8.6. COMPARISON OF WATER REABSORPTION FROM DLH AND CD

Use the results of Exercise 8.4 to make quantitative comparison of the flow of water out of the descending limb of Henle's loop with the flow of water out of the collecting duct when ADH is present. Recall that we made the approximation that the latter flow is small in comparison with the former.

8.7. A MORE COMPLETE MODEL

How are the equations of the model changed when the flow of water out of the collecting duct is not neglected? (Hint: This water has to be picked up by the peritubular capillaries.)

Solve the equations of this more accurate model under the assumption that c^* is given and compare the results with those of section 8.5. In particular, show that

1. The interstitial fluid is slightly more *dilute* when the kidney is in the concentrating mode than when it is in the diluting mode.

2. The approximation of neglecting the flux of water out of the collecting ducts gets better and better as $c^*/c(0) \to 0$.

9

Muscle Mechanics

In this chapter, we consider some macroscopic and microscopic aspects of how muscles work.

9.1 The Force–Velocity Curve

An important property of muscle is the relationship between the *force* P which it generates and the *velocity* V of its shortening. Observations of muscles under tension reveal a relationship between force and shortening speed like that shown in Figure 9.1.

The force–velocity curve characterizes a muscle in a constant contractile state. Such a state can be achieved in an isolated muscle by rapid, repetitive electrical stimulation. In life, a constant contractile state is achieved by sending a steady stream of nerve impulses to signal the muscle to contract. A muscle in a constant contractile state (and within a certain range of lengths) shortens at a rate that is determined by the load (or force) at the ends of the muscle. It is this relationship that is depicted in Figure 9.1.

Two important points on the force velocity curve are its intercepts with the coordinate axes: When $P = 0$, the muscle shortens at its maximum velocity, $V_{\max}$. As the load is increased, the velocity of shortening gets smaller, until the *isometric force*, P_o, is reached, at which the muscle cannot shorten ($V = 0$).

A.V. Hill was first to notice that the experimental force–velocity curves are closely fitted by an equation of the form

$$V = b(P_o - P)/(P + a) \qquad (9.1.1)$$

where P_o is the isometric force, and a and b are constants that can be determined from the experimental data. To do this, we first determine P_o as the force at which contraction does not occur. Then data points (V_n, P_n) are observed for $n = 1, \ldots N$. The relation

$$(P + a)V = b(Po - P)$$

is linear in the parameters a and b and it is therefore one to which the method of least squares (see Section 1.1.3) can be applied. In particular, it shown there how a and b can be chosen so that

$$\Sigma[(P_n + a)V_n - b(P_o - P_n)]^2$$

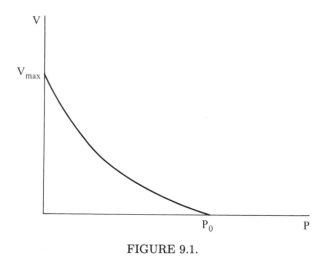

FIGURE 9.1.

is minimized. This gives the "best" estimate of a and b from data. $V_{\max}$ can be determined by setting $P = 0$ in (9.1.1) and solving for V. The result is

$$V_{\max} = bP_o/a. \qquad (9.1.2)$$

The remainder of this chapter is devoted to a derivation of the form of Hill's force–velocity curve from a microscopic theory of muscles.

9.2   Cross-Bridge Dynamics

We now turn to a microscopic description of the contractile process in skeletal muscle. As indicated in Figure 9.2, the *sarcomere* is a basic unit of muscle function. This contains the *thick filaments* and *thin filaments* that slide past each other during the process of contraction. These filaments do not change length during contraction of the muscle, but their relative motion is brought about by the *cross-bridges* between them.

The cross-bridges are armlike projections from the thick filaments that connect and disconnect with the thin filaments in response to the composition of their chemical environment. Immediately after such a connection is established, a chemical reaction occurs that puts the cross-bridge into a strained configuration. The cross-bridge then pulls the thin filament toward the center of the sarcomere. A second chemical reaction leads to breakage of the cross-bridge connection to the thin filament. This is referred to as the *cross-bridge cycle*.

The smooth contraction of the sarcomere is brought about by the combined activity of the entire cross-bridge population. The events of attachment and detachment occur essentially at random and independently in different cross-bridges. The chemical environment of the sarcomere governs the mean

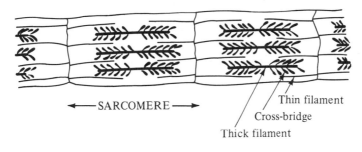

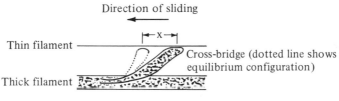

FIGURE 9.2.

attachment and detachment rates. On the other hand, the motions of the attached cross-bridges are coordinated since these motions are determined by the sliding velocity of the filaments. The sliding velocity is the same for all of the cross-bridges in a sarcomere.

As the sliding of the filament carries the cross-bridge away from its initial configuration, the strain of that configuration is relieved, and the force on the thin filament is reduced. At higher velocities of shortening, this happens faster. Thus, the muscle develops smaller forces at higher velocities of shortening. This effect explains, qualitatively at least, the form of the force–velocity curve. Such considerations can be made quantitative as follows.

We assume that an attached cross-bridge has an equilibrium configuration in which it exerts no force on the thin filament, and we let x denote the displacement from this equilibrium configuration measured along the thin filament. Let $p(x)$ be the force on the thin filament when the displacement of the cross-bridge is equal to x. A specific formula for $p(x)$ is introduced later, but for now we note that $p(0) = 0$, since $x = 0$ is the equilibrium configuration of an attached cross-bridge, and that $p(x)$ is an increasing function of x. Let n_o be the number of cross-bridges in a half sarcomere. All of these cross-bridges are effectively in parallel (their forces add), and all of the half sarcomeres are effectively in series (their lengths add). Accordingly, the force on the ends of the muscle if all cross-bridges are attached and had displacement x would be $n_o p(x)$.

In general, the different cross-bridges have different values of x, and we describe the cross-bridge population by the *population-density function* $u(x)$ defined by

$$\int_{x_1}^{x_2} u(x)\, dx = \quad \text{fraction of bridges with displacement } x$$

$$\text{such that } \quad x_1 < x < x_2. \tag{9.2.1}$$

We take the point of view that the quantity x is only defined for an attached bridge. The total fraction of bridges that are attached is given by

$$U = \int_{-\infty}^{\infty} u(x)\, dx < 1. \tag{9.2.2}$$

The force on the ends of the muscle, P, is also given by an integral over the cross-bridge population:

$$P = n_0 \int_{-\infty}^{\infty} p(x)\, u(x)\, dx. \tag{9.2.3}$$

To understand this formula, think of $n_o\, u(x)\, dx$ as the number of bridges with displacements in an interval of length dx near x. Then $n_o p(x) u(x) dx$ is the force exerted by the bridges in this interval, and the integral over all x gives the total force.

The cross-bridge *cycle* (attachment, sliding, detachment) is described in quantitative terms as follows: We assume that all cross-bridges form their attachments in a certain configuration $x = A > 0$. The rate of attachment of new bridges is proportional to the number of bridges that are available for attachment at any given time. In a half sarcomere, this number is $n_o(1 - U)$. Thus, we assume that the rate of formation of new bridges in a half sarcomere is $\alpha n_o(1 - U)$, where the constant α is called the *rate constant* for attachment. Note that α has units of time^{-1}.

Attached cross-bridges move with the thin filament. Thus, an attached cross-bridge satisfies the equation

$$dx/dt = -v$$

where v is the shortening velocity of the thin filament relative to the thick filament. From the anatomy of the sarcomere and the arrangement of the sarcomeres in the muscle (Figure 9.2), we conclude that $v = V/2N$ where V is the macroscopic velocity of shortening for the muscle as a whole and where N is the number of sarcomeres that are connected in series to make up the muscle.

Finally, we assume that the rate of detachment of cross-bridges is independent of their configuration x. Thus, the rate that bridges break is proportional to the number of attached bridges. The constant of proportionality is denoted by β. The parameter β also has units of time^{-1}, and is called the rate constant for bridge detachment. If we restrict attention to those bridges that have x in some particular interval, say (x_1, x_2), then the number of such bridges (per half sarcomere) is

$$n_0 \int_{x_1}^{x_2} u(x)\, dx$$

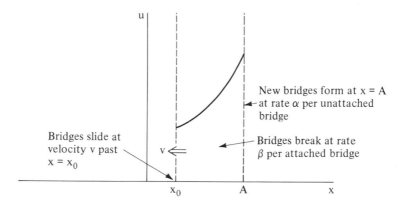

New bridges form at x = A
at rate α per unattached
bridge

Bridges slide at
velocity v past
x = x$_0$

Bridges break at rate
β per attached bridge

x_0 A   x

FIGURE 9.3.

and the rate at which these bridges break is

$$\beta\, n_0 \int_{x_1}^{x_2} u(x)\, dx.$$

The total rate of detachment is $\beta\, n_o\, U$.

We can now derive an equation for the cross-bridge population density $u(x)$. Our key assumption is that this population is in a steady state. Since cross-bridges are formed at $x = A$ and are moved by sliding in the direction of decreasing x, we have $u(x) = 0$ for $x > A$.

Consider the population of bridges that have x in the interval $x_o < x < A$ where x_o is any value of x such that $x_o < A$ (see Figure 9.3). New bridges enter this population by the process of attachment that occurs at the rate $\alpha\, n_o(1 - U)$. Bridges leave this interval in two ways: First, they break at the rate

$$\beta\, n_0 \int_{x_0}^{A} u(x)\, dx.$$

Second, they slide across the lower boundary at $x = x_o$. The rate of this last process is $v n_o u(x_o)$ since v is the velocity of sliding and $n_o u(x_o)$ is the density (number per unit length) of bridges at $x = x_o$.

Because the cross-bridge population is in a steady state, the three rates that we have considered must balance. This gives the equation

$$\alpha(1 - U) = \beta \int_{x_0}^{A} u(x)\, dx + v\, u(x_0) \tag{9.2.4}$$

where we have divided through by the common factor n_o.

This integral equation for u can be used to derive both a differential equation that holds for $x < A$, and a boundary condition that holds at $x = A$. To get the differential equation, differentiate (9.2.4) with respect to x_o. The result is

$$0 = -\beta\, u(x_0) + v\, (du/dx)(x_0). \tag{9.2.5}$$

Since x_o can be any value of x, this differential equation can be written more simply as

$$v\,(du/dx) = \beta\,u. \tag{9.2.6}$$

The solutions of this equation have the form

$$u(x) = u(A)\exp(\beta(x - A)/v). \tag{9.2.7}$$

The constant $u(A)$ in (9.2.7) is not yet determined, however. Note that (9.2.7) applies only when $x < A$. On $x > A$, we have $u(x) = 0$.

To derive an equation for $u(A)$, we go back to (9.2.4) and set $x_o = A$ (strictly speaking, we let $x_o \to A^-$). The result is

$$\alpha(1 - U) = v\,u(A) \tag{9.2.8}$$

which asserts that new bridges are carried away from $x = A$ as fast as they are formed.

Unfortunately, (9.2.8) does not quite determine $u(A)$ since U is still unknown. Integrating (9.2.7) from $-\infty$ to A, we find that

$$U = \int_{-\infty}^{A} u(x)\,dx = v\,u(A)/\beta. \tag{9.2.9}$$

This gives another relationship between U and $u(A)$, so we can solve (9.2.8) and (9.2.9) as a pair of linear equations in these two unknowns. The result is

$$U = \alpha/(\alpha + \beta) \tag{9.2.10}$$

$$u(A) = \alpha\beta/(v(\alpha + \beta)) \tag{9.2.11}$$

so that for $x < A$,

$$u(x) = \alpha\beta\exp(\beta(x - A)/v)/[v(\alpha + \beta)] \tag{9.2.12}$$

and $u(x) = 0$ if $x > A$. This result is plotted in Figure 9.4 for two different sliding velocities v. Note that the total number of attached bridges n_oU is independent of v. For low v, the bridges are clustered near $x = A$, whereas for large v they are more spread out in the direction of negative x.

Having determined the behavior of the cross-bridge population, we can now calculate the force–velocity curve. From (9.2.3), we have that

$$P = [\alpha\beta/(v(\alpha + \beta))]\int_{-\infty}^{A} n_op(x)\exp(\beta(x - A)/v)\,dx. \tag{9.2.13}$$

To proceed further, we need to know $p(x)$, the force exerted by a single cross-bridge in configuration x. The simplest hypothesis would be $p(x) = kx$, which would mean that the cross-bridge acts like a linear spring. As shown in Exercise 9.1, this hypothesis leads to a linear force–velocity curve. Here, we assume that

$$p(x) = p_1(\exp(\gamma x) - 1) \tag{9.2.14}$$

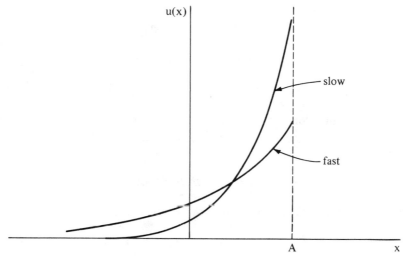

FIGURE 9.4.

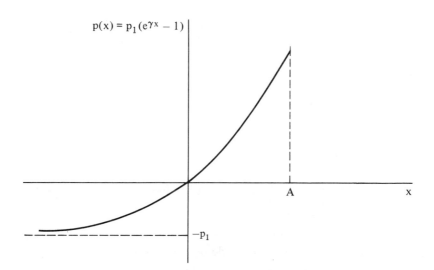

FIGURE 9.5.

which is plotted in Figure 9.5.

Substituting this expression in (9.2.13) and evaluating the integral {see Ex. 9.2}, we get

$$P = [\alpha \, n_o p_1/(\alpha + \beta)][((e^{\gamma A} - 1) - (\gamma v/\beta))/(1 + (\gamma v/\beta))] \qquad (9.2.15)$$

which is a formula for the force-velocity curve. Solving for $\gamma v/\beta$, we get

$$\gamma v/\beta = [(\alpha \, n_o p_1/(\alpha + \beta))(e^{\gamma A} - 1) - P]/[P + \alpha \, n_o p_1/(\alpha + \beta)]. \qquad (9.2.16)$$

This has the same form as the empirical force–velocity curve in equation (9.1.1). Since the velocity V at the ends of the muscle is related to v according to $V = 2Nv$, we have as before

$$V = b(P_o - P)/(P + a) \qquad (9.2.17)$$

where the constants P_o, b, and a are now given by the formulae

$$P_o = (\alpha \, n_o p_1/(\alpha + \beta))(\exp(\gamma A) - 1) \qquad (9.2.18)$$

$$b = 2N\beta/\gamma \qquad (9.2.19)$$

$$a = \alpha \, n_o p_1/(\alpha + \beta). \qquad (9.2.20)$$

Since $V_{max} = bP_o/a$, we also have

$$V_{\max} = (2N\beta/\gamma)[\exp(\gamma A) - 1] = 2N\beta A[\exp(\gamma A) - 1]/(\gamma A). \qquad (9.2.21)$$

In short, we have derived the empirical force–velocity curve from a particular model of cross-bridge dynamics, and we have determined the relationship between the microscopic properties of the model cross-bridges and the macroscopic constants of the muscle. The formula for the isometric force can be explained by the observation that all of the attached cross-bridges have the configuration $x = A$ when $v = 0$. Thus, the force exerted by each of these bridges is $p(A) = p_1(\exp(\gamma A) - 1)$. Since the number of attached bridges is $\alpha n_o/(\alpha + \beta)$, P_o is given by Equation (9.2.18).

The maximum velocity of shortening is determined by setting $P = 0$. This means that the negative forces exerted by the cross-bridges with $x < 0$ balance the positive forces exerted by the cross-bridges with $x > 0$. The velocity at which this occurs is independent of the overall size of the cross-bridge population. Thus, V_{max} is independent of αn_o.

It is interesting to contrast the behavior of P_o and V_{max} with respect to the parameter β, which is the rate of detachment of cross-bridges. Increasing β *decreases* P_o by decreasing the number of attached bridges. When β increases, $V_{\max}$ *increases*, however, because rapid detachment prevents most bridges from sliding into negative values of x where they would oppose shortening. A muscle with high β is fast but weak; a muscle with low β is slow but strong.

9.3 Annotated References

There are many aspects of muscle mechanics that could not be covered in this introductory Chapter. The reader who would like a more comprehensive treatment of the subject will find it in:

> Huxley, A.F.: *Reflections on Muscle* (The Sherrington Lectures XIV). Princeton University Press, Princeton, NJ, 1980.

The classic paper on the force–velocity curve of muscle is that of A.V. Hill:

> Hill, A.V.: The heat of shortening and the dynamic constants of muscle. *Proceedings of the Royal Society B* **126**, 136–195, 1938.

The idea that the mechanical behavior of muscle could be explained in terms of the dynamics of the cross-bridge population was introduced by A.F. Huxley:

> Huxley, A.F.: Muscle structure and theories of contraction. *Progress in Biophysics* **7**, 255–318, 1957.

The particular cross-bridge theory used in this Chapter is similar to Huxley's but not quite the same. It was introduced in the Ph.D. thesis of H.M. Lacker and is further discussed in the following reference:

> Lacker, H.M. and Peskin, C.S.: A mathematical method for the unique determination of cross-bridge properties from steady state mechanical and energetic experiments on macroscopic muscle *Lectures on Mathematics in the Life Sciences* **16**, American Mathematical Society, Providence, RI, 1986, 121–153.

Exercises

9.1. LINEAR FORCE–VELOCITY CURVE

Show that the assumption $p(x) = kx$ leads to a linear force–velocity curve.
Do this in two ways:

1. By substituting $p(x) = kx$ in (9.2.13) and evaluating the integral. Try
   integration by parts

2. By noticing that $p(x) = kx$ is a limiting case of an exponential spring.
   That is,

$$p_1(\exp(\gamma x) - 1) = p_1\gamma x(\exp(\gamma x) - 1)/\gamma x \to kx$$

   as $\gamma \to 0$, $p_1 \to \infty$, but with $p_1\gamma = k$. Having made this observation,
   take the corresponding limit in (9.2.17) through (9.2.21) and check that
   your result agrees with part 1 of this Exercise.

9.2. DERIVATION OF THE FORCE–VELOCITY CURVE

Write out the derivation of (9.2.15).

9.3. SUPER-ISOMETRIC FORCE

When a force greater than the isometric force is applied to a muscle, the muscle
stretches at a velocity that depends on the applied force. Calculate the force–
velocity curve for stretch making the same assumptions that were made in this
chapter. Remarks: Treat stretch as a *negative* velocity of shortening ($v < 0$).
Cross-bridges still form at $x = A$, but now they are carried into the region
$x > A$ by the sliding process. Thus, $u = 0$ for $x < A$, and the equation that
replaces 9.2.4 is

$$\alpha(1 - U) = \beta \int_A^{x_0} u(x)\,dx - v\,u(x_0).$$

Starting from this equation, repeat the derivation that led to the force–velocity
curve and see what you get. Sketch the behavior of the force–velocity curve
for positive and negative velocities of shortening on a single graph.

9.4. WHY MUSCLES YIELD AT LARGE SUPER-ISOMETRIC
FORCES

The force–velocity curve for stretch computed in Exercise 9.3 predicts infinite force at a finite velocity of lengthening. This is very unrealistic. In fact,
muscles *yield* when the applied force is greater that 1.8 P_o. That is, there is a
maximum force that the muscle can sustain. To explain this kind of behavior,
modify the cross-bridge model by assuming that bridges inevitably break if

they reach a configuration $x = B$, where $B > A$. This has no effect on the force–velocity curve for shortening, but it does influence the force–velocity curve of lengthening, since all of the integrals now extend over the interval (A, B) instead of (A, ∞).

1. Derive a formula for the force–velocity curve of lengthening for this model. Express your result in terms of the dimensionless variables $P^* = P/P_o$, $v^* = \gamma v/\beta$ and in terms of the dimensionless parameters $r^* = \alpha/\beta$, $A^* = \gamma A$, and $\omega = \gamma(B - A)$.

2. Show that your result reduces to the force-velocity curve calculated in Exercise 9.3 when $B = \infty$.

3. Make a quantitative plot of v^* as a function of P^* for both shortening and lengthening when $r^* = A^* = \omega = 1$.

4. Explain why the muscle has a finite maximum force when B is finite and why this force becomes infinite as $B \to \infty$.

5. On your graph, it should look as though the force–velocity curves of lengthening and shortening join up smoothly at $v^* = 0$, even though these curves are described by different formulae. How many derivatives of the two curves actually match at $v^* = 0$?

9.5. QUICK STRETCH

A muscle is shortening at velocity V and force P. Suddenly the muscle is stretched by an amount ΔL. The stretch is too sudden for any cross-bridges to break or for any new cross-bridges to form during the stretch.

1. What happens to the cross-bridge population $u(x)$ during the stretch?

2. What happens to the force P?

3. How could such experiments be used to check the hypothesis that $p(x) = p_1(\exp(\gamma x) - 1)$?

10

Biological Clocks and Mechanisms of Neural Control

A clock has three main parts: an oscillating system, such as a pendulum, spring, or electrical circuit; a source of energy; and a trigger mechanism or escapement that connects the energy source to the oscillator. A clock's face presents the oscillator's output in some useful way.

Biological clocks have the same ingredients. For example, a nerve cell's membrane is an oscillator, the energy is supplied by the cell's metabolism, and the trigger mechanisms are controlled ionic channels in the membrane. The result is a cycle of membrane voltage whose phase can be viewed as a hand moving on a clock face.

Natural rhythms of approximately 1 day were observed in animals by Aristotle, and it is now known that all living things have a variety of rhythms [1]. These rhythms are sometimes driven by external signals, like the interval of light seen by an animal each day (photoperiod), or by internal mechanisms, like circuits in the brain stem that control heart beat or breathing [2], [3]. In addition, internal and external timers can interact to cause interesting behavior, like that observed in foraging activity by voles who are nocturnal when the light interval is long and diurnal when the light interval is short each day [4], [5].

The timers studied here are nerve cells, or *neurons*. They set the beat. Muscles and glands act like filters and actuators that scale time by averaging neuron output, and physiological observable, like regular respiration or regular hormone cycles result. In this chapter, we consider some interesting aspects of clocks and of neurons that have suggested good experiments. In turn, the experiments suggest refinements in the model, etc. This process gives some insight into how neural networks can be studied using mathematical models.

Biological clocks are rarely isolated. They all operate in a common chemical bath, and there are many electrical, chemical and physical connections between them. It is difficult to grasp the complications of living with many clocks running at different rates, but the mathematical methods derived in this chapter can help. We will see how one clock can modulate another and how small networks of neurons can interact to control breathing.

A mathematical theory of clocks is developed first, and it is shown how some electrical circuits that are similar to neurons can be constructed.

The underlying oscillator in neuronal processes is the alternating flow of ions, charged molecules of sodium and potassium, through the nerve cell's membrane. We review some important aspects of cell membranes that were developed in Chapter 7, and then we look more carefully at the structure of neurons. In contrast to our earlier work, we pay special attention here to the dynamics of the membrane potential. In particular, neurons can transmit information by modulating their firing frequency, much like FM radios, and we focus on this aspect in our discussion of neurons as timers. Electronic circuits are described here that simulate important timing aspects of neurons.

In Section 10.2, we present clear physiological evidence that there is a phase-locked relation between oscillating stimulation and response in neuronal tissue. In 10.3 we derive the VCON model which is a constructible electronic circuit. We show that it has phase-locked responses to oscillatory stimulation, similar to neuronal tissue. Physiological data also show that neural circuits involve excitatory and inhibitory connections. This is described in Section 10.4, and it is shown how VCONs can be connected in excitatory and inhibitory ways. Based on this work, we are in a position to leap into neural circuit modeling. The results are electronic circuits that mimic neural activity, which, for example, can be used as analog control circuits in robots. The model circuits may even tell us something about how neurons and our brains work. We study in detail the von Euler mechanism for respiration control during exercise. Several other important neural circuits are studied in the Exercises.

10.1   A Theory of Clocks

Clocks are devices that we grow up with, and we do not think much about them. We learn to tell time by the location of the big and little hands on a clock face, and we ignore the fact that the numbering system is discontinuous. We also expect that the hands proceed at a uniform rate throughout a day.

There are many timing devices in our lives that distort these features. Body timers move rapidly through parts of a day or month and slowly through other parts. A similar effect on a wall clock would be to accelerate the hands during the morning and to slow them down during the afternoon. Or, we could use unequal spacings of the marks around the edge of a 24-hour clock to tell body time, morning times being spaced closer and afternoon ones farther separated while the hands move at uniform rates. The discussion of clocks here accounts for changes in the rate of advance of the hands. First, some mathematical descriptions of clocks are derived, then later, applications to phase-resetting experiments are discussed.

10.1.1   THE CLOCK ON THE WALL

Time can be measured using an arbitrary scale around a clock face's edge: minutes like on a wrist watch or radians as shown in Figure 10.1. We choose radians for mathematical convenience. If θ denotes the angle ("time") shown on the clock, then θ might increase proportional to solar time, or it might change at some other fixed rate. For example, we could have $\theta = \alpha t$ where

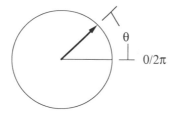

FIGURE 10.1. A clock face that has a single hand with time measured in radians.

t indicates Greenwich Mean Time, say measured in seconds, and α denotes the number of radians moved per second. It is more convenient to write this mathematical description of the clock as a differential equation

$$d\theta/dt = \alpha \qquad (10.1.1)$$

which indicates that the rate of change of θ is α. Note that the units of θ are radians and those of α are radians/time. Because of this, we refer to α as being a *frequency*, and θ is referred to as a *phase variable*. Given the value of θ, the coordinates of the hand are $x = R\cos\theta, y = R\sin\theta$ where R is its length. Note that this clock goes counter-clockwise (unless $\alpha < 0$).

This model (10.1.1) is referred to as a *simple clock*. A simple harmonic oscillator gives further insight to the model. Consider the equation $d^2u/dt^2 + \omega^2 u = 0$, which models small oscillations in a pendulum or the voltage of an LC-circuit [6]. All solutions have the form $u = A\cos(\omega t + \phi)$ where A and ϕ are arbitrary constants. If we set $u = A\cos\theta$, then we get that $d\theta/dt = \omega$. Thus, the harmonic oscillator is equivalent to a simple clock since the problem can be reduced to a single equation for the phase θ, provided $A \neq 0$. In fact, most oscillators can be reduced to phase equations except in certain singular cases [7] {see Ex.10.1}.

10.1.2   PHASE RESETTING: A RUBBER HANDED CLOCK

What time is it at the North Pole? We are imprinted with the solar clock, but it is not so clearly defined at the North Pole. The same question resides in the clock on the wall. Namely, if we can look only at the exact center of the clock, then we cannot tell the time. Similar timing problems have been observed in various biological timers, including neurons, and for guidance we turn to some interesting experiments on phase resetting.

Phase resetting experiments have helped in many ways to uncover biological rhythms. For example, a hamster kept in a cage under controlled conditions of light and dark, say having 16 hours of light and 8 hours of darkness each day (which we denote by L:D = 16:8), will use its exercise wheel at regular times during the dark period. When the light–dark conditions are changed to L:D = 0:24, the hamster continues to run at regular intervals like before, but slightly shifted to a shorter "day." The timing of the exercise period can be

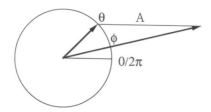

FIGURE 10.2. Perturbation of a rubber-handed clocks.

changed, either slowed down or accelerated, by briefly shining a bright light on the animal at various times during its activity period (see [4] [6]).

A modification is made to a simple clock to enable our study of phase resetting. Let us consider a *rubber-handed clock*. By this we mean a clock like that depicted in Figure 10.1, but whose hand has the following unusual properties:

1. left undisturbed, the hand's motion is described by the differential equation

$$d\theta/dt = \alpha.$$

2. if the hand is pulled or crushed and then released, it returns instantly to its original shape, but in the direction it points when let go.

3. except, if the hand is crushed to the center of the clock, it stays there.

A typical experiment is shown in Figure 10.2 where the hand is pulled A units to the right, then released. The clock is reset from phase θ to phase ϕ.

We see from this that tugging or crushing the hand leads to a resetting of the clock's phase. Thus, we can perform some *phase-resetting experiments* on this device.

Our principal experiment consists of shocking the system at various times by moving the hand A units horizontally and then releasing it. We record the phase at which the hand is moved (θ), the amplitude of the perturbation (A), and the new phase that the clock is reset to (ϕ).

The result is surprisingly complicated, but a short calculation gives theoretical predictions for the outcomes of these experiments. If the clock is at phase θ, then the hand extends from the origin (center of the clock) to the point $(\cos\theta, \sin\theta)$ on the clock's edge (we take the length of the hand at rest to be 1). Moving the clock's hand horizontally A units changes it into a hand extending from the origin to the point $(A + \cos\theta, \sin\theta)$, where we release it. The change of angle is $\Delta(A, \theta) = \theta - \phi$, and this difference can be determined using the law of cosines. In particular, the dot product of the two vectors defined by the two hand locations is the product of their lengths and the cosine of the angle between them:

$$(\cos\theta, \sin\theta) \cdot (A + \cos\theta, \sin\theta)$$
$$= \cos\Delta(A^2 + 2A\cos\theta + 1)^{1/2}$$

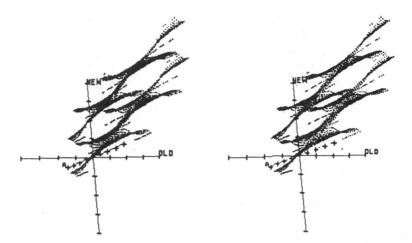

FIGURE 10.3. A cross-eyed sterographic randition of the phase-resetting surface for the rubber-handed clock. Here θ = old phase and ϕ = new phase. (Reprinted by permission from Oxford University Press.)

The result is a formula for $\cos \Delta$:

$$\cos \Delta = (1 + A \cos \theta)(A^2 + 2 A \cos \theta + 1)^{-1/2}.$$

We can solve this for the new phase ϕ by inverting the cosine, but some care is needed to do this. For example, if $\theta = \pi$ and $A = 1$, then the right hand side of this formula has the "value" 0/0! This reflects the fact that if the hand is crushed to the center of the clock, we cannot read the time.

It is interesting to plot the results of our analysis. We write

$$\phi = \theta + cos^{-1}((1 + A \cos\theta)(A^2 + 2 A \cos \theta + 1)^{-1/2}) \qquad (10.2.1)$$

being careful to invert the cosine correctly, and we plot ϕ as a function of θ for several fixed values of A. Some samples are plotted in Figure 10.3.

As simple as this model is, results quite similar to these have been found experimentally in resetting of *exercise wheel activity* by hamsters and voles and *eclosion* of fruit flies (drosophila). A version of formula (10.2.1) has been used in a variety of ingenious ways by A. Winfree (see [8]).

The connection between the rubber-handed clock and real biological timers in plants and animals is a difficult one to make. Little is known about the physiology of, say, foraging activity by small mammals, and for the present we settle for the phenomenological model that the rubber-handed clock provides.

On the other hand, this model suggests an experiment to determine whether neurons can be quenched by a timely shock. Such an experiment was performed by R. Guttman [9], and the result is that a correctly timed pulse can shift the neuron from repetitive firing to rest. Similar results have been found in heart muscle [10]. Heart muscle cells are driven by neurons, and their pacemaker activity can similarly be destroyed. This is believed to be a cause of kinds of cardiac *fibrillation*.

We proceed with the clear understanding that phase equations are relevant to the timing behavior of oscillators, but they do not tell the whole story. In particular, amplitude quenching like that discussed here is not accounted for. These are cases where oscillations are forced into singular situations where timing is destroyed. In those cases, reduction to phase variables alone is not appropriate {see Ex. 10.2}.

10.1.3 MODULATED CLOCKS

A *simple clock* is driven by a motor that moves its hand at a constant rate α. The human body does not always perceive time in this way. In fact, it happens that a neuron's base driving frequency can be *modulated* by many things, among them solar time brought into the body through sunlight. The mathematical model

$$d\theta/dt = \alpha + f(2\pi t/1440),$$

where f has period 2π, shows how a simple clock could be modulated by an external signal. When t increases through one day by minutes (1440 minutes per day), then the modulation f passes through one full cycle. This equation indicates that the hand moves in an irregular way throughout the day. For example, this clock is accelerated ($f > 0$) or slowed down ($f < 0$) in response to the time of day, perhaps due to sunlight or temperature.

An observable might be a point (cos θ, sin θ) where now $\theta = \alpha t + F(t)$ where $dF/dt = f(2\pi/1440)$.

The phase resetting experiments can be written in terms of a simple clock namely,

$$d\theta/dt = \alpha + \delta(t - t^*)\Delta(A, \theta^*)$$

where δ is the Dirac delta function indicating a impulse at time $t = t^*$, and $\Delta(A, \theta^*)$ is the phase shift in Equation (10.2.1) observed due to a perturbation A at (old) phase θ^*, provided A and θ^* are not a singular combination. Here $t^* = \theta^*/\alpha$. The result is that

$$\theta(t) = \alpha t + \Delta(A, \theta^*)H(\theta - \theta^*)$$

where $H(\theta) = 1$ if $\theta > 0$ and it is zero otherwise.

Clocks can also be modulated by other clocks, and we will eventually relate neurons to simple clocks, but first we turn to experimental work done on nerve membranes {see Ex. 10.3}.

10.2 Nerve Cell Membranes

Hodgkin and Huxley [11] studied a patch of membrane taken from the giant axon of a squid. They modeled the potassium and sodium ion channels using a simple electrical circuit. Unfortunately, their model turns out to be difficult to use to make predictions and suggest experiments. Because of this various caricatures of the membrane patch have been formulated and studied. These are fill-and-flush models where charge accumulates in some device representing the membrane and is eventually released. Such models have been based on simple switches, tunnel diodes, transistors, and voltage controlled oscillators [6].

Since we are focusing on timing aspects of cells, we review certain data obtained in [12], and we take a certain view toward modeling based on modern integrated circuitry.

Alternating flows of various ions through membranes establish electrical currents that carry information. In this section, we recall from Chapter 7 some of the physical properties of these membranes.

10.2.1   CELL MEMBRANE POTENTIAL

Recall from Section 7.3 that an electrical potential is established across a membrane by having different concentrations of chemical species on either side. If a semipermeable membrane separates two regions of space that have concentrations (mass/volume) of ions, say C_i inside and C_o outside, then a short calculation shows that

$$qE = k\mathbf{T}\log(C_o/C_i)$$

where q is the charge on each ion, E is the resulting potential, k is a gas constant, and T is the absolute temperature. This leads to the *Nernst equation*:

$$C_o/C_i = \exp(qE/k\mathbf{T})$$

or

$$E = -(k\mathbf{T}/q)\log(C_i/C_o).$$

This equation shows how to calculate the membrane potential once the ion concentrations inside and outside are known.

The important ions that maintain the cell membrane potential are sodium (Na^+) and potassium (K^+). Each ionic species has associated with it a membrane potential that is maintained by relative impermeability of the membrane to the other species. For example, if the membrane is impermeable to Na^+, then a high concentration of K^+ inside the cell will force K^+ ions through the membrane by molecular diffusion and electrical repulsion. This continues until the electrical potential balances the concentration gradient. At equilibrium, the Nernst equation shows that

$$E_K = (k\mathbf{T}/q)\log(C_o^K/C_i^K) \sim -75mV.$$

This is referred to as the *potassium resting potential*. Similarly, if the membrane is impermeable to K^+, but not to Na^+, we have

$$E_{Na} = (k\mathbf{T}/q)\log(C_o^{Na}/C_i^{Na}) \sim 55mV$$

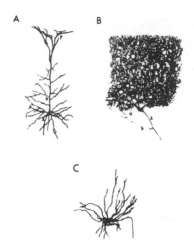

FIGURE 10.4. A. Pyramidal cell. B. Purkinje cell. C. Spinal motoneuron. (Reprinted from drawings of Ramon Y. Cajal, by permission from Consejo Superior de Investigaclones Científicas.)

which is called the *sodium resting potential*. The total cell potential changes in response to the opening and closing of ion channels in the membrane. This was described in Section 7.4.

There is a substantial jump in passing from experiments done for a small patch of axon membrane to behavior of an entire nerve cell. In fact, neurons remain largely unknown. There are many different kinds of neurons, and how they work is slowly emerging. Still, an important part of the neuron is its spike generator which creates action potentials; the cell output is, in major part, created by spikes causing the release of chemical neurotransmitters outside the cell. Because of this, we reduce our view of the whole cell to its spike generator.

Several sketches of neurons are shown in Figure 10.4.

The principal interest here is in the neuron's hillock region of the cell body at the base of an axon. This region can generate electrical activity in the form of voltage pulses called action potentials. A pulse can propagate along the axon away from the hillock region to its terminus in a synapse. When a pulse arrives at a synapse, it causes the release of chemical signals, called neurotransmitters, outside the cell. The neurotransmitter can then interact with the membrane of another neuron to move it toward firing if it is an excitatory neurotransmitter, like acetylcholine, or inhibit it from firing if it is an inhibitory neurotransmitter, like GABA [13].

Neuron membranes at rest are relatively impermeable to Na^+. Therefore, the observed potential is near E_K. When excited, Na^+ channels open rapidly and the membrane potential approaches E_{Na}. The K^+ channel opens more slowly, but eventually the membrane potential returns to near E_K. This is shown in Figure 10.5 where the sign of voltage is positive relative to outside.

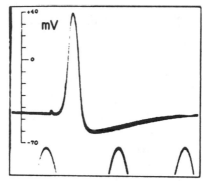

FIGURE 10.5A. Plot of an action potential from Hodgkin and Huxley. (Reprinted by permission from Nature, vol. 144 pp. 710-711. Copyright ©1939 MacMillan Magazines, Ltd.)

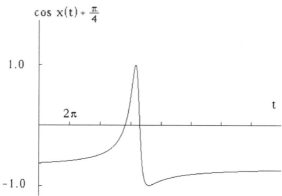

$$x' = 1. + \cos x$$
$$x(0) = \pi + 0.1$$

FIGURE 10.5B. $\cos(\theta + \pi/4)$, where $d\theta/dt = 1 + \cos\theta$.

The precise mechanisms that control these channels remain unknown.

A neuron can fire repetitively, but the actual physiology of repetitive firing is more complicated than studied here.

Let $V(\theta)$ denote a nerve cell's membrane potential with phase θ. V is the waveform of an action potential as in Figure 10.5A, but we see in Figure 10.5B that $V(\theta) = \cos\theta$ gives a profile similar to an action potential when its phase is correctly determined {see Exercise 10.4}. For a typical neuron that is firing repetitively, $\alpha = 2\pi/(3.0E - 3 \text{ sec})$ (recall that the notation $3.0E - 3 = 3.0 \times 10^{-3}$), and for it an action potential has a period of 3 msec. We therefore write

$$d\theta/dt = 2\pi/(3.0 \times 10^{-3})$$

and we observe the membrane potential to be $\cos 2\pi t/(3.0 \times 10^{-3})$. When t increases by 3.0E-3 seconds, one full action potential is created. Thus, embed-

TABLE 10.1. Guttman's Data

Frequency Response of Squid Axon

Stimulus Intensity ($\mu A/cm^2$)	Stimulus Frequency (Hz)								
	20	40	60	80	100	120	140	160	180
34.2	0	0	.113	.5	.12	0			
37.8	0	0	.5	.5	.5	.18	0		
41.4	0	.87	.77	.5	.5	.41	0		
45.0	0	1	1	.53	.5	.5	.33	.12	0
50.4	0	1	1	.67	.5	.5	.38	.33	.11
57.6	0	1	1	.79	.5	.5	.5	.32	.33
62.1	.64	1	1	.92	.5	.5	.5	.34	.34
70.2	1	1	1	1	.67	.5	.5	.47	.33
72.9	1	1	1	1	.67	.5	.5	.5	
77.4	1	1	1	1	.75	.5	.5	.5	
82.8	1	1	1	1	1	.67	.5	.5	.5
86.4	1	1	1	1	1	.67	.5	.5	.5
90.0	1	1	1	1	1	.75	.5	.5	.5
113.4	1	1	1	1	1	1	.67	.5	.5
148.5	1	1	1	1	1	1	1	.75	.5
220.5	1	1	1	1	1	1	1	1	1
351.0	1	1	1	1	1	1	1	1	1

ded in a repetitively firing neuron is a simple clock. To simplify the notation, we take $V(\theta) = \cos\theta$ {see Exercise 10.4}.

10.2.2 GUTTMAN'S EXPERIMENTS

Guttman, et al. [12], stimulated a preparation of squid axon membrane similar to Hodgkin and Huxley's with oscillatory voltages of various amplitudes and frequencies. A stimulus of frequency μ and amplitude A was applied, and the response of the patch was recorded. The response was usually observed to be a regular voltage oscillation having an easily determined frequency, say ω. The results are presented in terms of the frequency response ratio ω/μ, as described in Table 10.1. A plot of some of these data (a transect at $\mu = 120$ Hz) is presented in Figure 10.6.

The intervals over which $\omega/\mu = 1$ are sets of stimulation amplitudes for which the neuron is *locked onto* the forcing frequency! This is referred to as 1:1 *phase locking* in the electrical engineering literature, and it is an important aspect of many designed electrical circuits [14]. Note that there are significant combinations of stimulus parameters for which interesting fractional responses are observed, especially $\frac{1}{2}$, $\frac{2}{3}$, $\frac{3}{4}$, etc.

There are many other neuronal systems that are known to phase-lock. These

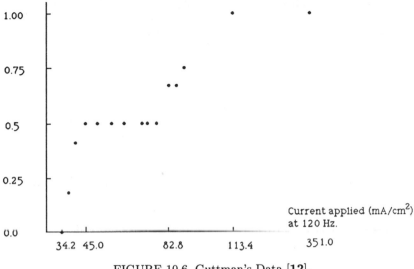

FIGURE 10.6. Guttman's Data [12].

include the abdominal ganglion of Aplysia californicus (sea slug) and the
thoracic stretch receptors in Procambarus clarkii (crayfish) [15],the auditory
nerve fibers of the squirrel monkey [16], the lateral eye of Limulus (horseshoe
crab) [17], breathing and stride in humans [18], and foraging behavior in Microtus montanus (montane vole)[5]. The model of a spike generator that we
derive next will have phase-locking properties similar to Guttman's observations [12]

10.3   VCON: A Voltage-Controlled Oscillator Neuron Model

Electrical circuits are described in terms of the physical quantities of voltage
(V) and current (I). The ideas of voltage and current are not intuitive since
they cannot be directly observed by us without special instruments. However,
one can think of voltage as being a pressure that pushes electrons (charges)
and of current as being a measure of the electron flow. These can be measured
precisely by voltmeters and ammeters, respectively.

Although electrical circuits are the basis of radios, TVs, and computers and
their peripherals, they are also important in understanding how our bodies
work. As we have seen, most nerve activity is electrical. Ionic currents through
membranes and across synaptic gaps are dominant physical properties of neuron networks including the brain. Modeling these aspects of cells can take
advantage of recent developments in integrated circuits. Happily, electrical
engineers have taken the view of many circuits as being clocks, and they have
designed many of them to have models that are similar to the simple clock

model in order to simplify the design of larger circuits. This section describes an integrated circuit that keeps time and has many of the features already noted here for neuronal tissue. To do this, it is not necessary to study electrical circuit theory in any depth, but only to understand the input/output relations of particular circuits.

10.3.1 VOLTAGE-CONTROLLED OSCILLATORS

There are a number of brilliantly designed modern integrated circuits that are remarkably simple to describe, although the details of them are quite complicated. Several are used here.

The basic circuit element used in the neuron model presented later is an oscillator, much like a simple clock, whose frequency is modulated or controlled by an input voltage. There are many kinds of *voltage-controlled oscillators,* but we denote a generic one by VCO and depict it by the graph

$$V_{in} \rightarrow VCO \rightarrow V(\theta)$$

where the input voltage V_{in} and the output voltage $V(\theta)$ are related in a somewhat complicated way, but the main variable being measured is the *phase* of the output voltage, θ.

Current is ignored at this level of modeling VCOs, and the model is described in terms of the input and output voltages alone: The output of the VCO is an oscillatory function V of the phase $\theta(t)$. V is a fixed wave form, depending on the chip used. Commercially available VCOs put out waveforms V that are square waves, triangular waves, or sinusoidal waves. For example, $V(\theta) = \cos \theta$ indicates that the output is sinusoidal. However, if V is a square wave, then the VCO output is like a *van der Pol* relaxation oscillator that has played a central role in the theory of neurons since the 1920s. To fix ideas, we take $V(\theta) = \cos \theta$.

By design of the circuit, the phase θ is related to the controlling voltage by the differential equation [14]

$$d\theta/dt = \omega + V_{in}(t)$$

where the constant ω is called the VCO *center frequency.* This equation can be solved by integrating it directly:

$$\theta(t) = \theta(0) + \omega t + F(t)$$

where $\theta(0)$ is the initial phase and $dF/dt = V_{in}(t)$. Thus, the larger ω or V_{in} is, the faster will θ increase, and so the faster will $\cos \theta$ oscillate. Therefore, a VCO is like a simple clock that can be modulated by an input (controlling) voltage. Note that if V_{in} is constant and equal to $-\omega$, then $\theta(t)$ and so $\cos \theta$ are constant.

10.3.2 PHASE COMPARATORS AND A MODEL SYNAPSE

Another useful electronic device is a *phase comparator*. It compares oscillatory voltages and it puts out a signal depending on the two input phases. This output might be used as the controlling voltage of a VCO, as we see in the next section. The simplest phase comparator is a device that simply multiples two rectified voltages: Two voltages $V_+(\psi)$ and $V_+(\theta)$ put into the phase comparator, the first having phase ψ and the second with phase θ give an output that is the product of $V_+(\theta)V_+(\psi)$. Here we denote by V_+ the positive part of V:

$$
\begin{aligned}
V_+ &= (V + |V|)/2 \\
&= \max(V, 0) \\
&= V \text{ if } V > 0, \quad \text{but it is zero otherwise.}
\end{aligned}
$$

If V is a periodic function, then the product $V_+(\theta)V_+(\psi)$ has a rich Fourier series that includes terms of the form $\cos(\theta - \psi)$. The structure of this Fourier series is an important aspect of phase-locking [6].

An action potential is generated in the cell body of a neuron and propagates out along the axon toward the synapse. When it arrives, it can cause vesicles in the synapse to contract and so release *neurotransmitters* into the synaptic gap between this cell and another. The neurotransmitters diffuse across the gap and interact with a dendrite or with the cell body. If they are *excitatory neurotransmitters*, then they increase the dendrite's membrane potential and so move the receiving cell toward generating its own action potential. If they are *inhibitory*, then they retard the receiving cell from generating an action potential.

A synapse can be roughly modeled in the following way: Let V denote the membrane potential of the first cell. If it exceeds a threshold, say $V = 0$, it will cause the release of neurotransmitters and so cause a change in the receiving cell's membrane potential, which we denote by U.

In our simplified study here, we *ignore*

1. the diffusion of neurotransmitters

2. the dendritic structure of the receiving cell

3. the propagation time along the axon.

Roughly, our model is one of the spike generator driving a very short axon that terminates in an electrical synapse attached directly to the receiving cell's body.

We describe the active part of V as its positive part, since this is part of it that exceeds the synapse's threshold.

The influence of the arriving signal on the receiving cell's membrane potential U is limited by physiological limits of nerve cell membranes. In particular, a membrane can support only a limited potential (see Section 7.5). Therefore, an *excitatory synapse* results in adding the two potentials up to a limit above which, for practical purposes, the response is constant. An *inhibitory synapse* (i.e., one having inhibitory neurotransmitters) is modeled by taking the difference of the U and V_+ down to a lower limit, below which the response is constant. Therefore, we denote the response of the synapse by

$$\tanh(U + A\,V_+)$$

where tanh is a convenient sigmoid-shaped function and the sign of A denotes the polarity of the synapse ($A > 0$ means an excitatory synapse, $A < 0$ denotes an inhibitory one), the amplitude of A indicates the strength of the synapse and tanh clips the combined potential to physiological limits [**6**].

If the sending cell has membrane potential $V(\psi)$ and the receiving cell's membrane potential is $V(\theta)$, then the output from the synapse to the hillock region is taken to be

$$\tanh(V(\theta) + V_+(\psi)).$$

This function is periodic of period 2π in θ and ψ, and it has a Fourier series. In particular, if $V(\theta) = \cos\theta$, then this Fourier series is quite rich since most of its coefficients are not zero, and among them is the term $\cos(\theta - \psi)$. Because of this, we see that the model synapse behaves quite like the phase comparator described earlier {see Exs. 10.5, 10.6}.

We will simplify this model by replacing $\tanh(U + V_+)$ by $U + V_+$.

10.3.3   VCON: A MODEL SPIKE GENERATOR

The next step in developing our model neuron is to describe a neuron's spike generator. There is evidence that the cell body behaves quite like a voltage-controlled oscillator, although presenting this evidence requires work that is outside the scope of this book (see [**6**] for details). However, a brief description begins with the work of Hodgkin and Huxley on nerve membranes. They derived an electrical circuit model of squid axon membranes in 1952. Subsequent work has shown that many facets of that circuit are reproduced by a *van der Pol relaxation oscillator* or *multivibrator*, which are primitive forms of a voltage-controlled oscillator. Predictions made from studies of the van der Pol oscillator led to further experiments on squid axons by Guttman et al., who uncovered many interesting timing properties that nerve membranes have. Among these are rich phase-locking properties described earlier in Table 10.1 and Figure 10.6.

The voltage controlled oscillators described earlier provide a way to mimic these timing properties using only simple clocks and thereby facilitating our understanding. In taking this approach, we lose track of the individual ion channels in the neuron's membrane, but we rely on the experimental corroboration of using VCOs for its ultimate justification.

In our model, we attempt to describe only spike generation in the cell, and some aspects of interaction between such spike generators. The goal is to provide a simple model to study phase-locking. Strictly speaking, we are

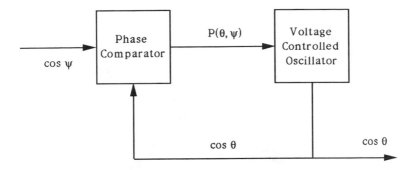

FIGURE 10.7. VCON: a voltage-controlled oscillator model of a neuron.

modeling the *hillock region* at the base of an axon of the cell body where action potentials are generated as being a VCO, and its output is our model's membrane potential.

The VCON model combines the cell body's output with the input from impinging synapses and feeds this back into the cell body as a controlling voltage. Figure 10.7 shows the equivalent circuit.

If the input voltage has the form $\cos\psi$ where ψ is given and the VCO's output is $\cos\theta$, then the mathematical model of this circuit is simply

$$d\theta/dt = \omega + P(\theta, \psi)$$

which has the form of a simple clock modulated by the input and its own potential. The modulation is more complicated now than before, but the model is quite easy to understand. Some properties of the VCON model are uncovered in the next section and in Exercise 10.6.

10.3.4 PHASE-LOCKING PROPERTIES OF A VCON

Let us perform Guttman's experiment on the VCON model. This entails solving the problem

$$d\theta/dt = \omega + \cos\theta + A\cos_+ \mu t$$

where $A\cos_+ \mu t$ is the forcing potential. We can simulate Guttman's experiments by solving this problem for large time and calculating the ratio $P = x(t)/\mu t$. The results are described in Figure 10.8.

It is remarkable that such a simple model can reproduce phase-locking plateaus similar to those observed for a complicated membrane system. Using a richer phase comparator in the VCON results in richer combinations of phase locking [**19**] {see Exs. 10.7, 10.8}.

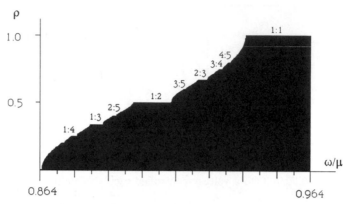

FIGURE 10.8. VCON rotation number $A = 1.1, \mu = 1/6$.

10.4   Neural Control Networks

Simple clocks and the VCON model can lead to some understanding of how neurons respond to various inputs and how they can be control devices in the body. We first describe network notation, and then an example of a neural control system. The example describes a simple network that is implicated in a variety of physiological control systems, including human respiration.

10.4.1   NETWORK NOTATION

The graph

$$N_1 \rightarrow^+ N_2$$

indicates a network of two neurons in which N_1 has an *excitatory synapse* impinging on N_2.

The VCON analog of this network can be modeled using the VCO phases of each. Let θ_1 and θ_2 denote these phases, so the model membrane potentials of the cells are $\cos\theta_1$ and $\cos\theta_2$, respectively. The network is then modeled by the differential equation

$$\begin{aligned} d\theta_1/dt &= \omega + \cos\theta_1 \\ d\theta_2/dt &= \omega + \cos\theta_2 + A\cos_+\theta_1 \end{aligned}$$

where A is a positive constant. We have taken the center frequencies of each of these neurons to be the same, although in general, they are different.

The network

$$N_1 \rightarrow^- N_2$$

describes an *inhibitory synapse* from N_1 to N_2. The model is the same except that now A is a negative constant.

10.4.2   VON EULER'S RESPIRATION CONTROL MECHANISM

Human breathing is believed to be controlled by a small network of neurons in the brain stem that generate signals to inspiratory and expiratory muscles in the rib cage and on the diaphragm [2].

The pattern generator that controls respiration is not yet known, but an interesting suggestion about it is made by von Euler [20]. Whereas it is known that the control of respiration is more complicated than this simple mechanism, the von Euler mechanism is a building block useful in constructing models closer to real data. We will study the von Euler model by formulating a VCON version of it.

In this system two VCONs drive the diaphragm, one up and one down. The *inspiratory* VCON (phase θ_{in}) inhibits the *expiratory* VCON (θ_{out}), and it in turn can be inhibited by a VCON (θ_m) that models *stretch mechanoreceptors* driven by the diaphragm during deep breaths. The *diaphragm* is modeled as being a simple linear mass-spring system.

This example illustrates how firing on a time scale of milliseconds can cause regular oscillations on a much longer time scale (seconds in this case) through interaction with an inertial system. Similar neural networks might be involved in *hormone* levels in the blood, *activity/rest* cycles, and a variety of other physiological rhythms.

THE DIAPHRAGM AS A LINEAR MASS-SPRING SYSTEM

The *diaphragm* is attached to the bottom of the rib cage in humans, and it plays a central role in breathing. Muscles pulling it down cause breathing in, and natural restoring forces supplemented by muscles pulling it up cause exhalation, although expiratory muscle activity is thought to be more passive than inspiratory. The diaphragm has significant inertia because the stomach, liver, and other heavy objects are attached to it.

Additional complications result from the three dimensional structure of the diaphragm and the ways in which muscles are attached to it.

We view the diaphragm as being a piston that is moved up and down by *actuators* (muscles). The model describes the mass, resistance, and restoring force on the diaphragm as well as the transduction of neuron firing into muscle contraction that acts like an external forcing of the system.

The model of such a linear mass-spring system is a differential equation for the deflection of the diaphragm from rest. Let D denote the deflection, with $D > 0$ indicating inspiration (down in humans). Then D can be determined by solving the equation

$$m \, d^2D/dt^2 + r \, dD/dt + k \, D = F$$

where m is the mass, r is the coefficient of resistance, k measures the restoring force, and F is the external force applied to the piston. F will account for inspiratory and expiratory VCON activity and for external force applied to the diaphragm due to running {see Ex. 10.9}.

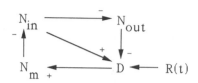

FIGURE 10.9. von Euler's mechanism where $R(t)$ is an external force applied to D by running: $R(t) = A \cos \sigma t$

Evaluating the data used in this model is difficult. For example, the mass of the stomach changes with drinking and eating, so m is not constant. Also, exact values for r and k are not known. Despite all of these drawbacks, the model is useful because it bears out von Euler's prediction that the mechanism will sustain regular oscillations in D.

Once the external force F is known, we can find D by solving this equation. However, the external force depends indirectly on the deflection D because feedback from breathing modulates the firing of the controlling neurons, as we see next.

This linear mass-spring system can be easily simulated using an RLC electrical circuit {see Ex. 10.9}.

A MECHANISM FOR PATTERN GENERATION

We model the von Euler mechanism by a single *inspiratory VCON* (N_{in}), a single *expiratory VCON* (N_{out}), and a single *mechanoreceptor VCON* (N_m). These have phases θ_{in}, θ_{out} and θ_m, respectively.

Firing of the inspiratory neuron causes the diaphragm to be pulled down. In response, when the diaphragm is deflected below a threshold, N_m is excited to fire and so inhibit N_{in}. When inhalation ceases, the restoring force of the diaphragm and the expiratory muscles start its return. The cycle then repeats itself.

The mechanism is described in Figure 10.9.

This network is easily modeled using VCONs. Let θ_{in} denote the firing phase of N_{in}, etc. Then the network is described by the equations

$$
\begin{aligned}
d\theta_m/dt &= 3.0 - 4.0 \cos \theta_m + 10.0 D_+ \\
d\theta_{in}/dt &= 3.0 - 2.0 \cos \theta_{in} - 4.0 \cos_+ \theta_m \\
d\theta_{out}/dt &= 2.5 - 2.0 \cos \theta_{out} - 4.0 \cos_+ \theta_{in} \\
50.0 \, d^2 D/dt^2 &+ dD/dt + D = F.
\end{aligned}
$$

In this circuit, 3.0 is the inspiratory neuron's firing frequency in the absence of external modulation {see Exercise 10.10}.

It only remains to determine what the external force is acting on the diaphragm. We model F simply by taking

$$
F = 5.0 \tanh(\cos_+ \theta_{in} - \cos_+ \theta_{out} + A \cos \sigma t)
$$

where A is a transduction constant describing the force applied to the diaphragm by external forcing due to running at step frequency σ. tanh is used to clip forces to physiological limits.

A numerical solution of this model is presented next.

SIMULATION OF RESPIRATION

The respiration model derived in the preceding section is quite complicated, but it is easy to solve on a computer. Figure 10.10 shows the results of two simulations. In the first, the model is solved for $R(t) = 0$. In Figure 10.10B, it is solved for $R(t) = \cos t/2.0$.

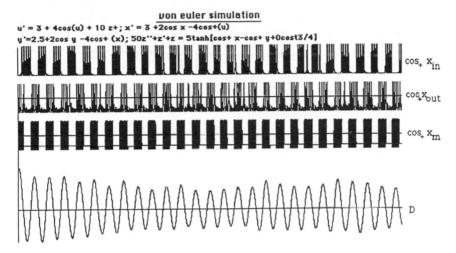

Next, we consider the model when we run with $A = 1.0$ and step frequency $\sigma = 0.5$. The result is shown in B.

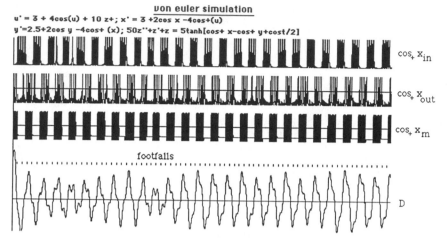

FIGURE 10.10B. Running and breathing. In this case there are 2 strides for every three breaths.

Respiration while running is quite interesting, and recent work by Bramble [18] has shed new light on synchronization between breath and stride in runners. Our simulation here shows three breaths for each two strides (left footfall to left footfall) {see Ex. 10.10}.

DISCUSSION OF RESPIRATION

von Euler's mechanism is easy to simulate using VCON models. It is not so easy to do using Hodgkin–Huxley's model or various fill-and-flush simplifications of it. Although the results in Figure 10.10 look promising, they only lay a basis for further research in respiration. This model is one step in an iterative procedure that uses experiments to motivate models and models to suggest new experiments. As this procedure converges, new insights are gained. The respiration model illustrates this nicely. von Euler's network is quite robust, as our crude modeling and simulation indicates.

Finally, we note that in the respiration model, the diaphragm is an oscillatory system that is driven by energy sources (the neuron potentials). The escapement in this case is the threshold of stimulation of the mechanorepectors that the diaphragm traverses. Thus, this higher order rhythm has the ingredients of a clock described at the start of this chapter.

10.5   Summary

There is clear physiological evidence that neurons phase-lock onto oscillatory stimulation and that inhibitory and excitatory connections between neurons create important firing patterns that are used to control body systems. Motivated by this, we presented the VCON circuit, which is about the simplest system that will exhibit phase-locking. In fact, the development of VCONs is based on work done in teaching courses that led to this book. The exercises give some neural circuits other than von Euler's where VCONs have been used. The first, called the atoll oscillator {see Ex. 10.11}, is a simple pair of VCONs that produces bursts. In fact, they illustrate firing behavior that occurs on two time scales. The second circuit is the tonotope {see Ex. 10.12}. This describes a signal fanned out onto a network of VCONs that is graded by center frequencies. This shows how a temporal signal can be converted into a spatial pattern of firing fibers, and then after correlations between outputs, how a characteristic response can be educed. Finally, a model for how the brain might focus attention one among many competing stimuli is described in Exercise 10.13.

This work reminds us of the caution we expressed in the Foreword. We have pruned away features of neurons that are not needed to produce the kinds of outputs we seek. In doing so, we have dropped many of the known aspects of neurons. Still, the results give a constructible circuit that exhibits the desired behavior.

The VCON is a constructible electronic circuit, it has a mathematical model that is easy to understand, and it lends itself to computer simulation. Hopefully, this work will enable the reader to keep up with developments in neuroscience as they emerge by trying to reproduce new observations using VCON analog circuits

10.6   Annotated References

1. R. R. Ward, *The living clocks*, A. A. Knopf, New York, 1971.

2. A.J. Vander, J.H. Sherman, and D.S. Luciano, *The mechanisms of body function*, McGraw-Hill, 1975.

3. S.W. Kuffler, and J.G. Nicholls, *From neuron to brain*, Sinauer, Sunderlund, MA, 1976.

   An accessible general neurophysiology text.

4. K. Hoffman, *Splitting of circadian rhythms as a function of light intensity*, Biochronometry, pp 134-151, National Academy of Sciences, Washington DC, 1971.

5. C. Rowesmitt, et al., *Photoperiodic induction of diurnal locomotor activity in Microtus montanus, the montane vole*, Can. J. Zool. **60** (1982), 2798–2803.

6. F.C. Hoppensteadt, *An introduction to the mathematics of neurons*, Cambridge Univ. Press, Cambridge, UK, 1986.

   Many of the topics of this chapter are developed here in greater depth.

7. J.K. Hale, *Ordinary differential equations*, J. Wiley, New York, 1969.

8. A.T. Winfree, *The geometry of biological time*, Springer–Verlag, New York, 1980.

9. R. Guttman, S. Lewis, and J. Rinzel, *Control of repetitive firing in squid axon membrane as a model for a neurone oscillation*, J. Physiol. **305** (1980), 377–395.

10. A.T. Winfree, *When time breaks down*, Princeton Univ. Press, 1987.

11. A.L. Hodgson, and A.F. Huxley, *A quantitivative description of membrane current and its application to conduction and excitation of nerve*, J. Physiol. **117** (1952), 500–544.

    This classic paper started the Hodgkin–Huxley theory.

12. R. Guttman, L. Feldman, and E. Jakobsson, *Frequency entrainment of squid axon membrane*, J. Membrane Biol. **56** (1980), 9–18.

13. H.C.Tuckwell, *Introduction to theoretical neurobiology*, Vols 1 and 2 Cambridge Univ. Press, New York, 1988.

14. P. Horowitz and W. Hill, *The art of electronics*, Cambridge Univ. Press, New York, 1989.

    An excellent reference on modern electronic circuits.

15. D.H. Perkel, J.H. Schulman, T.H. Bullock, G.P. Moore, and J.P. Segundo, *Pace maker neurons: effects of regularly spaced synaptic input*, Science **163** (1964), 61–63.

16. J.E. Rose, J.F. Brugge, D.J. Anderson, and J.E. Hind, *Phase-locked responses to low frequency tones in single auditory nerve fibers of the squirrel monkey*, J. Neurophysiol. **30** (1967), 769–793.

17. C. Ascoli, M. Barbi, S. Chillemi, and D. Petracchi, *Phase-locked responses in the Limulus lateral eye*, Biophysical J. **19** (1977), 219–240.

18. D. Bramble, and D.R. Carrier, *Running and breathing in mammals*, Science **21** (1983), 251–256.

19. F.C. Hoppensteadt, *Intermittent chaos*, PNAS, (USA) **86** (1989) 2991–2995.

20. C. von Euler, *Central pattern generation during breathing*, Trends in Neuroscience, Nov. 1980, 275–277.

21. F.C. Hopensteadt, *The searchlight hypothesis*, J. Math. Biol., **29** (1991), 689–691.

22. H.D. Patton, A.F. Fuchs, B. Hille, A. Scher, and R. Steiner, *Textbook of physiology*, Vol 1, W.B. Saunders, 1989.

This is a most important reference for work in physiology.

23. F. Crick, *Function of the thalamic reticular complex: the searchlight hypothesis*, PNAS, (USA) **81** (1984), 4586–4590.

Exercises

10.1 CLOCKS

a. Solve the equation $d\theta/dt = \alpha$ for $\theta(t)$ and plot the points using polar coordinates $x = \cos\theta(t)$, $y = \sin\theta(t)$ in the xy-plane.

b. Consider two independent clocks having phases θ and ϕ. Solve the two equations $d\theta/dt = \alpha$ and $d\phi/dt = 1$ and plot θ and ϕ modulo 2π; that is, plot the results on a square in the $\theta\phi$-plane that has side 2π. Show that if α is a rational number, then the oscillators are synchronized, but if α is irrational, then they are chaotic relative to each other.

Plot the points with coordinates

$$
\begin{aligned}
x &= (1 + \cos\phi)\cos\theta \\
y &= (1 + \cos\phi)\sin\theta \\
z &= \sin\phi
\end{aligned}
$$

in the three-dimensional xyz-space as θ and ϕ range over the square $0 \le \theta, \phi \le 2\pi$. Show that this describes a torus.

Let θ and ϕ be the solutions of the differential equations above, and plot the corresponding trajectory on the torus. Time on the two independent clocks can be read simultaneously by using the toroidal clock face.

c. Consider a system of differential equations in polar coordinates ($r^2 = x^2 + y^2$ and $\theta = \tan^{-1} y/x$),

$$
\begin{aligned}
dr/dt &= r(1 - r) \\
d\theta/dt &= \alpha.
\end{aligned}
$$

Describe the solution of this system that starts at the point $r(0) = 0.01$, $\theta(0) = 0.0$. Find the simple clock among the solutions of this system for various choices of $r(0)$ and $\theta(0)$.

10.2. PHASE RESETTING

a. Derive formula (10.2.1).

b. Set $A = 1$ and plot all points (θ, ϕ) for which formula (10.2.1) is satisfied. Repeat this for several values of A. This calculation identifies singularities in the surface.

c. Perform the phase-resetting experiments using the model in Exercise 10.1.c. Note that if a pulse having amplitude near 1.0 is applied near $\theta = \pi$, then the resulting solution must spiral out for a long time before arriving near the circle $r = 1.0$. Interpret this for the timing that this clock provides.

10.3. MODULATED CLOCKS

a. Plot the values of $\cos(\alpha t + \Phi(t))$ where

$$d\Phi/dt = \cos(2\pi t/100.0)$$

for each of the values $\alpha = 1.0$ and $\alpha = 2\pi/100.0$.

b. Plot the solutions of the equation

$$d\theta/dt = \alpha + \delta(t - t^*)\Delta(A, \theta^*)$$

where $t^* = \theta^*/\alpha$ and Δ is given in formula 10.2.1.

10.4. VCON'S ACTION POTENTIAL

a. Reproduce Figure 10.5B. That is, using a computer solve the equation

$$d\theta/dt = 1 + \cos\theta$$

using various initial data. Plot $\cos(\theta + \pi/4), \cos\theta$, and $\cos(\theta - \pi/4)$.

b. Do the same for the equation

$$d\theta/dt = 1 + 0.006\pi + \cos\theta.$$

10.5. PHASE COMPARATORS

Construct contour plots for the following phase comparators (that is, find the values of θ and ψ [modulo 2π] for which $P = c$ for various choices of the constant c):

a. $P = \cos\theta + \cos_+ \psi$

b. $P = \cos_+ \theta \, \cos_+\psi$

c. $P = \tanh(\cos\theta + \cos_+\psi).$

In addition, in the first two cases, find the Fourier series of the function in terms of the two independent phase variables ϕ and ψ {see Ex. 4.10}.

10.6. VCONS

Derive the VCON model for the circuit in Figure 10.7 in each of the three cases in Exercise 10.5. In each case, plot $d\theta/dt$ versus θ and describe what the solutions do when there is no input.

10.7. PHASE-LOCKING SIMULATIONS FOR VCON

Reproduce the computer experiment described in Figure 10.8 in the three cases of phase comparators in Exercise 10.5.

10.8. PHASE-LOCKING ANALYSIS

a. Consider the system of two equations

$$dx/dt = \omega + \cos(x - y)$$
$$dy/dt = \mu.$$

Show that if $\mid \omega - \mu \mid < 1$, then $x - y \to C$, a constant, as $t \to \infty$. Deduce that $x \to \mu t + C$ and that $x(t)/y(t) \to 1.0$ for all such values of ω and μ. This is the simplest example of phase-locking.

b*. Consider the system of two equations

$$dx/dt = \omega + \cos(x - y) + \cos(2x - y)$$
$$dy/dt = \mu.$$

Show that if $\mid \omega - \mu \mid << 1$, then $x/y \to 1.0$ and if $\mid 2\omega - \mu \mid << 1$, then $x/y \to 0.5$. This can be done either using computer simulations as in the preceding exercise or by mathematical analysis.

10.9. LINEAR MASS-SPRING SYSTEMS

Model the equation of an RLC circuit

$$V_{in} \to \quad \text{Resistor (R)} \quad \to \quad \text{Inductor (L)} \quad \to \quad \text{Capacitor (C)} \quad \to \quad \text{Ground.}$$

Let V denote the voltage across the capacitor and use Kirchhoff's Laws to derive an equation for V. (Total voltage around any closed loop in a circuit is zero; total current into any point in a circuit is conserved.) We see that this equation has the same form as the one for the linear mass-spring model diaphragm, so an RLC circuit can be used to simulate such a linear mass-spring system.

10.10*. VON EULER'S MODEL

a. Simulate von Euler's neural circuit in Section 10.4.2 when $A = 0.0$. That is, reproduce Figure 10.10A.

b. Simulate von Euler's circuit when $A = 1.0$ for various choices of footfall frequency σ. Describe phase-locking between breathing and stride.

10.11*. THE ATOLL OSCILLATOR

Consider the system of two VCONs

$$dx/dt = 1.1 + \cos x - \cos_+ y$$
$$dy/dt = 0.01(1.0 + \cos y - 20.0 \cos_+ y).$$

Plot solutions of this system on the torus $0 \leq x < 2\pi$, $-\pi \leq y < \pi$. Show that the set of x and y for which

$$1.1 + \cos x = \cos_+ y$$

defines an atoll-like region; that is, the solutions move slowly around it, but rapidly outside and deep within it. Plot the solutions $x(t)$ and $y(t)$ versus t, and observe that the system puts out bursts of activity.

10.12*. A TONOTOPE

a. Acoustic signals are processed by various nuclei of neurons when their effect on the basilar membrane is passed on to the brain for processing. The tonotope is a typical processing unit in this pathway [22]. A simplified VCON version of a tonotope is described by an array of VCONs whose center frequencies are graded:

$$\frac{dx_j}{dt} = \omega_j$$

where $0 < \omega_o < \omega_1 < \omega_2 < \ldots < \omega_N$. To fix ideas here, let $\omega_{j+1} - \omega_j = 0.1$. A temporal signal, say $f(t)$, can be fanned out onto this array with the resulting system being

$$\frac{dx_j}{dt} = \omega_j - f(t)\cos_+ x_j.$$

Compute the solutions of this system when $N = 100$ and $f(t) = \cos_+ t$. Observe that the spatial pattern of output frequencies describes plateaus of phase-locking.

b. There are neural cells in the auditory system that correlate inputs. The VCON version of this is the simple model

$$\frac{dz}{dt} = \mu + \cos_+ x_k \cos_+ x_j.$$

The output is a voltage whose phase is

$$z(t) = \mu t + \int_0^t \cos_+ x_k(s) \cos_+ x_j(s)\, ds.$$

Thus, the output frequency of this circuit is

$$\mu + \frac{1}{t}\int_0^t \cos_+ x_k(s) \cos_+ x_j(s)\, ds$$

which is the correlation between the two input signals. Pass the output of the gradient system in part a through a layer of correlating cells:

$$\frac{dz_j}{dt} = \mu + \cos_+ x_j \sum_{k=1}^{N} A_{k,j} \cos_+ x_k$$

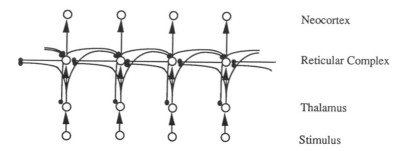

FIGURE 10.11. A thalamic reticular complex model circuit. ↑ denotes an excitatory synapse, $-\bullet$ denotes an inhibitory synapse.

where the $A_{kj} = 1$ for nearest neighbors ($| k - j | \leq 1$) and are zero otherwise.

Calculate the solution of this combined system and observe that the peaks of output from the correlating layer occur only where there is an interval of phase-locking.

If such neurons produce neurotransmitters in proportion to their firing frequency, then the correlation-cell production reflects the intervals of phase-locking in the first layer. Thus, the network performs a useful form of signal processing by converting a temporal signal $f(t)$ into a spatial distribution of firing frequencies or chemical concentrations. In either case, the output signal reflects the frequency spectrum of $f(t)$.

10.13*. ATTENTION: THE SEARCHLIGHT HYPOTHESIS

It has been proposed that the brain focuses attention on the most persistent among many competing stimuli using a circuit in the thalamus. We will model this using simplified VCON circuits. The result is an electronic circuit that will perform this feat.

The searchlight hypothesis [21], [23] conjectures that stimuli of various intensities arrive in the thalamus, and it passes only the most demanding stimulus to the neocortex for further processing. A hypothetical neural circuit was proposed in [23] that involves neurons of the thalamus (TH), the reticular complex (RC), and the neocortex (NC). A signal-excited thalamic cell excites a reticular complex cell, which feeds back inhibition to the thalamic cell in such a way that repetitive bursts are observed. The activity of the pair effectively inhibits other (nearby) RC cells and excites a single neocortical column structure.

A simplified model of this network uses VCONs. Our model is shown in Figure 10.11. The voltage phases are $x_0, \ldots x_N$, and $y_0, \ldots, y_N$, for RC and TH cells, respectively. The phases of the neocortical projections are $z_o, \ldots, z_N$. A VCON model for this network is

TABLE 10.2. Simulation of the Thalamic Reticular Complex Model with a Periodic
Array based on 15 VCON Pairs. (Each digit on the time line denotes 10 computa-
tional steps of size $2\pi/100.0$.)

Time   123456789012345678901234567890123456789012345678901234567676890
σ_0 .[0.01————————0.01][4.0–4.0].....................
NC_0 .....B.....................B..B...B......................
σ_1 ....[0.1————————————————————————0.1]
NC_1 .........B....B.............................B......B......
σ_2 ....[1.0————————1.0]....................
NC_2 ..................B..B..B......B...........................

$$\frac{dx_j}{dt} = 0.04(1 + \cos\ x_j + \tanh(5.0\cos_+\ y_j - 0.95\sum_{j'\neq j}(\cos_+\ x_{j'} + \cos_+\ y_{j'})))$$

$$\frac{dy_j}{dt} = 5.0(1 + \cos\ y_j + \cos_+\ \sigma_j t - \cos_+\ x_j)$$

$$\frac{dz_j}{dt} = 1 + \cos\ z_j + \cos_+\ x_j$$

for $j = 0, \ldots, N$. The constants in this network are chosen to have a ratio
of time scales approximately 100:1. The neocortex cells (not shown here) are
modeled by VCONs that are forced by $\cos_+ xj$.

  a. Simulate this system using $N = 15$, and suppose that the array is ex-
     tended periodically each 15 cells. Reproduce the results of solving this
     system (say, using a fourth order Runge-Kutta algorithm) as presented
     in Table 10.2.

  Initially, there is no stimulation to the network. At time $t = 2\pi/5.0$, a slow
stimulus of frequency $\sigma_0 = 0.01$ is presented to VCON 0, and eventually its
neocortex projection NC_0 fires a burst. Each **B** denotes a burst of approximately 10 action potentials. At time $t = 2\pi$ a stimulus of frequency $\sigma_1 = 0.1$
is presented to VCON 1, and its neocortex projection begins firing bursts and
NC_0 is silenced. Frequency $\sigma_2 = 1.0$ is applied to the third VCON at time
$t = 4\pi$, and frequency $\sigma_0 = 4.0$ is applied to the first VCON at time 6π.
The results are that the dominant stimulus takes over the network when it
is applied. There is only one spurious burst that appears on NC_2 at time
7π, otherwise the network passes forward only the dominant stimulus. In the
attention model, the interactions between neighbors is modulated by the tanh
term that clips the net input.

  b. Study the response of this network to various combinations of stimuli.

Answers for Selected Exercises

Chapter 1

1.2: The characteristic equation is $r^2 - ar - b = 0$ so

$$r_{\pm} = \frac{a \pm \sqrt{a^2 + 4b}}{2}$$

If the largest root is less than 1, then $R_n \to 0$. Otherwise, $r_+^{-n} R_n \to C > 0$. Find C by writing $R_n = Cr_+^n + B\ r_-^n$. Solve for B and C using the initial conditions. If $a = 0$, then the alternate-year classes are independent of each other.

1.4.a. Show that for $M \le 2$ there is no irregular behavior of solutions. If $M \ge 3$ it is possible. Carry out the histogram experiment in several of these cases.

1.4.b. Solutions approach constants for $r \le 3.0$. Above that there is a cascade of new periodic behavior, at each step the period being double what it was before. This ends at approximately $r = 3.57$, where the behavior becomes chaotic.

1.6.a. Show that $r_n \to 1$ as $n \to \infty$ by cobwebbing. Since $2^N \theta_0 = \theta_0 + 2\pi\ m$ for some integer m, we have that $\theta_0 = 2\pi m/(2^N - 1)$. Thus, for any integer m, this gives a periodic solution of the desired period. Obviously there are only 2^N choices for m.

1.6.b. For almost all choices of θ_0, the cells will be approximately equally occupied so $H \sim 1.0$. Therefore, the mapping is quite complicated.

1.7.a. Solve for P_n using back-substitutions and for $p(t)$ using separation of variables and estimate the difference between P_n and $p(nh)$.

1.7.b. If p is a solution of the equation $dp/dt = F(p)$, then if p is not strictly monotone there must be a point t^* where $dp/dt(t^*) = 0$, that is, where p changes from being strictly monotone. But at such a point $F(p) = 0$, so in fact, $p = p(t^*)$ is a solution of the equation! Since through any point there is at most one solution of this equation, it must be the constant one.

1.8. For example, if $S = K$, then the growth rate is exponential. This concentration is maintained if $\lambda = V/2$. Then $B = Y(S_o - k)$.

1.9. See [2] Chapter 1.

1.13. There are many solutions of the characteristic equation. Denote them by r_0, r_1, r_2, and order them by their real parts so that

$$r_0 > Re\ r_1 \geq Re\ r_2 \geq \ldots$$

Laplace's method shows that

$$B(t) = \sum A_k e^{r_k t} \sim A_0 e^{r)_0 t}.$$

Find r_0 using Newton's method. That is, define

$$f(r) = \int_0^\infty b(a)\lambda(a)e^{-ra}da - 1$$

and define approximations $R_o = 1.0$, and for $n = 1, 2, \ldots,$

$$R_{n+1} = R_n - \frac{f(R_n)}{f'(R_n)}$$

where $f' = df/dr$. Evaluate the first five of these numbers.

Chapter 2

2.8. Direct calculation shows that

$$\mathbf{P}^n = \left(\sum_{j=1}^{M} \lambda_j \mathbf{P}_j \right)^n = \sum_{j=1}^{M} \lambda_j^n \mathbf{P}_j.$$

As a result,

$$\mathbf{P}^n = \sum_{j=1}^{k} \mathbf{P}_j + \sum_{j=k+1}^{M} \lambda_j^n \mathbf{P}_j.$$

The terms in the second series $\to 0$ as $n \to \infty$ since $| \lambda_j | < 1$. The transition probability matrix for the Fisher–Wright chain in Section 2.3 is

$$\mathbf{P} = \begin{pmatrix} 1.000 & 0.000 & 0.000 & 0.000 & 0.000 \\ 0.316 & 0.422 & 0.211 & 0.047 & 0.004 \\ 0.0625 & 0.25 & 0.375 & 0.250 & 0.0625 \\ 0.004 & 0.047 & 0.211 & 0.422 & 0.316 \\ 0.000 & 0.000 & 0.000 & 0.000 & 1.000 \end{pmatrix}$$

Show that the eigenvalues of this matrix are $1, 1$, and three others that satisfy $| \lambda | < 1$. This can be done by direct calculation or using a computer to iterate the matrix to see what survives.

2.10. More generally, consider an M-allele genetic trait where the gene pool proportions are $p_j j = 1, \ldots, M$. Let $1 + \epsilon m_{ij}$ denote the fitness of the genotype $p_i p_j$. Show that

$$\frac{dp_j}{dt} = \epsilon(\overline{M_j} - \overline{M})p_j$$

where

$$\overline{M_j} = \sum_{i=1}^{N} m_{i,j} \quad \text{and} \quad \overline{M} = \sum_{j=1}^{N} \overline{M_j}.$$

This calculation follows directly from the definitions.

Chapter 3

3.2. In case $p = .9$, the distribution of survivors is mainly focused near $S = 0$. For $p = .4$, the distribution is bimodal with comparable frequencies in both modes, and in the last case the distribution is mainly based near $S = 4$.

3.3. a. Since $0 \le x_{n+1} \le x_n$, $\{x_n\}$ is a nonincreasing sequence that is bounded below. Therefore, it has a limit.

b. $\exp(-ay_n) = x_{n+1}/x_n \to 1$ from a. Therefore,

$$y_n = (1/a)\log(x_{n+1}/x_n) \to 0.$$

c.

$$
\begin{aligned}
x_n &= x_{n-1}\exp(-ay_{n-1}) = x_{n-2}\exp(-a(y_{n-1} + y_{n-2})) = \dots \\
&= x_0\exp(-a(y_{n-1} + \dots + y_0)).
\end{aligned}
$$

Since $z_n = (1-b)y_{n-1} + z_{n-1} = (1-b)(y_{n-1} + y_{n-2}) + z_{n-2} = \dots = (1-b)(y_{n-1} + \dots + y_0)$, we have that $x_n = x_0\exp(-az_n/(1-b))$.

d. As $n \to \infty$, $x_n + z_n = N - y_n \to N$, so $z_\infty = N - x_\infty$. Also $N = y_0 + x_0$, so

$$-\frac{az_\infty}{1-b} = -\frac{ax_0}{1-b}(1 + i - F)$$

f. When there are very few infectives ($y_0 \sim 0$) two branches of the equation for F cross when $T = 1$ at $F = 1$. This signals the fact that for $T < 1$, the realistic solution is $F \sim 1$ and for $T > 1$ the realistic solution is $F < 1$.

3.4. See reference [4], Chapter 3.

3.11.a. The expression on the right hand side of the equation for $I(t)$ can be expressed as an integral:

$$\frac{dI}{dt}(t) = r\frac{d}{dt}\int_{t-\tau}^{t} I(s)(N - I(s))\,ds$$

Integrating this gives the formula

$$I(t) = C + r\int_{t-\tau}^{t} I(s)(N - I(s))\,ds$$

where C is a constant. If $I(t) \to I^*$, then

$$I^* = C + r\,\tau\,I^*(N - I^*).$$

Solve this for I^*.

b. Linearize the equation about $I = I^*$: That is, set $I = I^* + \delta I$. Then δI satisfies the equation

$$\frac{d\delta I}{dt}(t) = r(N - 2\,I^*)(\delta I(t) - \delta I(t - \tau)).$$

Look for solutions of this equation in the form $\delta I(t) = e^{\lambda t}$. If such a term is to be a solution, λ must satisfy the characteristic solution

$$\lambda = r(N - 2I^*)(1 - e^{-\lambda \tau})$$

Show that all, except for $\lambda = 0$, of the solutions of this equation for λ satisfy $Re\ \lambda < 0$ where $Re\ \lambda$ denotes the real part of the (possibly) complex number λ. Deduce that all solutions approach I^*.

Chapter 4

4.2.c. If a three- and a four-period focus are on the same grid, the three-period waves will eventually drive into the four period focus and annihilate it.

4.11. Substitute $u = (x - y)/\sqrt{4Dt}$ in the integral and let $t \to 0^+$ in the result.

4.13. Substituting $f(g) = g + F(g)\,\delta\,t$ results in the formula

$$g_{m,n+1} = \lambda(g_{m+1,n} + g_{m-1,n} - 2\,g_{m,n}) + g_{m,n} + \delta t\, F(g_{m,n})$$

Dividing both sides by δt and assuming that $\lambda\frac{\delta x^2}{\delta t} \sim D$, we get

$$\frac{g_{m,n+1} - g_{m,n}}{\delta t} \approx D\frac{g_{m+1,n} + g_{m-1,n} - 2g_{m,n}}{\delta x^2} + F(g_{m,n}).$$

Therefore, passing to the limit δx, $\delta t \to 0$ gives the result.

Chapter 10

10.1.a. This trajectory describes a circle that is traversed each time t increases by $2\pi/\alpha$ units.

10.1.b. The solutions are straight lines on the square. When one runs off the top, it enters the bottom, directly below its exit point. Similarly for lines running off either side or the bottom: lines running off the left reenter at the right at the same level, etc. The slope of these lines is $1/\alpha$. If a is rational, then the lines eventually repeat themselves. Otherwise, the lines never come in contact in the future and the solutions will be dense in the square. This is another form of chaos, like that discussed in Chapter 1.

The points describe a torus, and if α is rational, say $\alpha = p/q$ where p and q are integers, then the points will trace out a curve on the torus that wraps p times in the θ direction and q times in the ϕ direction before closing up and repeating itself. If α is irrational, the trajectory will cover the torus.

10.1.c. The solution of this system of equations is

$$r(t) = r(0)/(r(0) + e^{-t}(r(0) - 1)), \theta(t) = \alpha t + \theta(0).$$

Therefore, the simple clock is on the circle $r(0) = 1$. The solution to be plotted is a spiral beginning at $r(0) = 0.01$, $\theta(0) = 0.0$ and spiraling out to the circle $r = 1$ as $t \to \infty$.

10.2.b. See [8], Chapter 10.

10.2.c. The singularity at $r = 0$ for the rubber-handed clock now expands into a hole. If the system is driven near the value $r = 0$, then the time taken to emerge from this area and reestablish timing will be longer than the life-span of the observer. Therefore, the amplitude dependence that is introduced in this model causes a larger area of disruption of timing.

10.6. Show that if ω is small, then the solutions tend to a constant, but if ω is large, they tend to infinity.

10.7. Use the forward Euler algorithm to solve the differential equations using a computer, and calculate and plot $x(t)/t$ for large t in each case. The forward–Euler method for solving a differential equation

$$dp/dt = F(p)$$

is to introduce a step-size h and approximations $p_n = p(nh)$. Then

$$p_{n+1} = p_n + h\,F(p_n)$$

Great care must be taken in using this formula. Although it is easy to use, it is quite limited in stability, so results may not be reliable. The Runge-Kutta method in Ex. 10.10 is more complicated but also more reliable.

10.8.a. Let $u = x - y$. Then $du/dt = \omega - \mu + \cos u$. From Exercise 1.7.b, u is monotone. If $\omega - \mu$ is small, then u approaches a constant c for which $\omega - \mu + \cos c = 0$. b. See [19], Chapter 10.

10.9. Let v denote the voltage across the resistor and let i denote the current through it. Then from Ohm's Law $v = R\,i$ where R is a constant that quantifies the resistance. From Henry's Law, we have that the voltage across the inductor is $L\,di/dt$. Finally, from Faraday's Law $i = C\,dV/dt$ where C measures the capacitance. The total voltage across the circuit is V_{in} and so we have from Kirchhoff's Law the balance equation $V_{in} = R\,i + L\,di/dt + V$. Equivalently,

$$LC\,d^2V/dt^2 + RC\,dV/dt + V = V_{in}.$$

10. 10–13. The fourth order Runge–Kutta algorithm solves an equation

$$dx/dt = f(t, x)$$

from (t_o, x_o) to $(t_o + h, x_1)$, by defining four values:

$$
\begin{aligned}
k_1 &= h\,f(t_o, x_o) \\
k_2 &= h\,f(t_o + h/2, x_o + k_1/2) \\
k_3 &= h\,f(t_o + h/2, x_o + k_2/2) \\
k_4 &= h\,f(t_o + h,\ x_o + k_3)
\end{aligned}
$$

then

$$x_1 = (k_1 + 2k_2 + 2k_3 + k_4)/6.$$

This is a "good" differential equation solver since $x(h) - x_1 = O(h^4)$. It is better to use a package that avoids some of the general pitfalls, but the fourth order Runge-Kutta method is simple and reliable if the solutions don't change too quickly.

10. 10.b. Introduce the phase of the diaphragm oscillation by rewriting the diaphragm equation using polar coordinates $r^2 = D^2 + (dD/dt)^2$ and $\psi = \tan^{-1}(dD/dt)/D$. Calculate the ratio $\psi/\sigma t$ for large t and plot the result for various values of σ.

Index